THE ANTIOXIDANT PRESCRIPTION

THE

ANTIOXIDANT

PRESCRIPTION

*How to
Use the Power
of Antioxidants
to Prevent Disease and
Stay Healthy for Life*

BRYCE WYLDE

Bsc, RNC, DHMHS, ND

RANDOM HOUSE CANADA

Krahn, Bruce, "Your Personal Low-Injury Antioxidant Exercise Plan," pages 200–12. Copyright © 2008 eBodi Inc.
Tapp, Teresa, "Wellness Workout," pages 213–22. Copyright © 2008.
Illustrations pages 206–12 reprinted with the permission of John Wiley & Sons Canada, Ltd., a subsidiary of John Wiley & Sons, Inc.

This publication contains the opinions and ideas of its author. It is intended to provide helpful and informative material on the subjects addressed in the publication. It is sold with the understanding that the author and publisher are not engaged in rendering medical, health, or any other kind of personal professional services in the book. The reader should consult his or her medical, health, or other competent professional before adopting any of the suggestions in the book or drawing inferences from it.

The author and publisher specifically disclaim all responsibility for any liability, loss, or risk, personal or otherwise, which is incurred as a consequence, directly or indirectly, of the use or application of any of the contents of this book.

LIBRARY AND ARCHIVES CANADA CATALOGUING IN PUBLICATION

Wylde, Bryce
The antioxidant prescription : how to use the power of antioxidants to prevent disease and stay healthy for life / Bryce Wylde.
Includes index.

ISBN 978-0-307-35585-0

1. Antioxidants—Health aspects. 2. Nutrition. I. Title.
RB170.W94 2007   613.2'86   C2007-903427-6

Printed and bound in the United States of America

10 9 8 7 6 5 4 3 2 1

To my wife, Kelly,
and my children,
Devin and Zaya—my life inspirations

CONTENTS

PART ONE: THE CAUSE OF ALL DISEASE

PART TWO: THE ACTION PLAN

PART ONE

—

THE CAUSE OF ALL DISEASE

CHAPTER 1

THE HUMAN HEALTH THRESHOLD

W e live in an era strangely cursed and blessed. We're increasingly surrounded by invisible dangers our great-grandparents could not have dreamed of. In fact, until recently, most of us hardly dreamed of them ourselves. But what we once suspected or heard rumoured, we now know for certain: Our air, our water, our food and many of the everyday objects we employ are a constant threat to our health and safety. And yet—and this is the blessed part—this same knowledge is our hope for a bright future for ourselves and for humanity at large.

The subject of human health is almost unimaginably vast, and our body's interactions with our surroundings are almost too complex to grasp. But in this book I'm going to zoom in and focus on the meaning of human health through the lens of a single natural phenomenon—I'm tempted to say "drama"—that plays out at a scale so tiny that ordinary microscopes cannot see its workings. There are villains in this drama but, as in any good story, these characters are dynamic. The fact is they often spend much of their time doing us a tremendous service. Even if we were able to round every one of them up and do them in, we'd be the ones to suffer in the end. That's why our task will be to understand them first, then deal with them wisely—perhaps I should say "humanely," since they're a necessary part of life.

This gang of wild molecules are called "free radicals." They're notorious these days and almost everyone has heard their name. Wanted posters appear regularly advertising methods for their capture and execution. I recently saw a video game devoted to a free radical mission. Yet a great deal remains to be conveyed about their behaviour and how we need to respond to that behaviour in order to stay healthy or to regain our health. Much of this *hasn't* been conveyed, in part because it's a breaking science story.

We hear even more these days about antioxidants, the molecules that neutralize free radicals and are supposed to be on our side in this battle. Are they the cure-alls they're made out to be? Are some antioxidants better than others? Can we swallow too many antioxidants? To establish your knowledge level about both free radicals and antioxidants before you carry on, take a moment to do the quiz you'll find in Appendix A.

In this book, I'm going to set out what you need to know about free radicals. I'm going to show you how and why free radicals lie at the root of all disease. I'm not just talking here about chronic diseases such as cancer, heart disease and allergies. I'm also talking about diseases that stem from infectious agents— bacteria, parasites and viruses. I'm then going to show how and why the antioxidant family of molecules works to offset the destructive impact of free radicals. Finally—based on the latest science—I'm going to show you how you can determine your own free radical and antioxidant levels and provide you with a simple prescription for supplements, diet and lifestyle that will balance your body's supply—or burden—of both these families of potent molecules.

THE SPROUTS AND I

I grew up in Toronto, Canada, a vegetarian and unvaccinated. I had the sort of mom who you could imagine treating the common cold by putting garlic between her son's toes, covering his feet with cold, wet socks to bring down a fever and maybe administering a twice-daily concoction of eye of newt and bat wing. In fact she did practise the cold-sock therapy and it turned out to be one of her good ideas. I also began every morning by swallowing ten vitamins and minerals. Our soaps and shampoos smelled of tea tree oil and were certainly free of harmful agents, though otherwise, er, not perfected. Junk food in my family was a sesame seed snap. Anything with sugar in it was considered to be deadly, and eating hotdogs was equivalent to swallowing poison. Birthday cakes were suspect. I went to school every day with a SoyPro, sprouts-and-tomato sandwich on thick German-style bread, the kind you could see the grains in. Needless to say, I kept this lunch hidden for fear of being ridiculed and possibly beaten. On occasion, I was able to "misplace" my lunch altogether and claim the peanut butter and jelly on soda crackers that the lunch room staff kept for those unfortunates who forgot their lunch.

Our family doctor, Dr. John McLean, was a chiropractor, a homeopath and a naturopath. Unless we were near death, my mother wouldn't bring us near the regular medical profession for fear its practitioners would fill us with antibiotics or surgically remove some vital organ we'd most certainly need later in life.

I should mention that my mother's view of the medical profession was very different then than mine is now.

When I grew older, I determined to become a clinical psychologist and spent a year volunteering at Toronto's Queen Street Mental Health Centre. My first day there was spent talking to a schizophrenic man in the patient library who was threatening to inject himself with Javex. After a year or so of similar efforts, I came to the realization that we were trying to make a difference for people who were little more than pharmaceutical overdose cases. One afternoon I stumbled across some old patient files in the facility's basement storage room. In them, I found evidence that, back in the early 1950s, some clinicians in that very institution had been incorporating homeopathic medicines with considerable success to treat mental illness. I decided that from that point forward, I'd try to make a real difference in the lives of others, not simply struggle to supersede the side effects of powerful drugs. It would be my mission to prevent people from getting to the point of incarceration in one of these hellholes.

I went to the Ontario College of Homeopathic Medicine in Toronto to study homeopathy, nutrition and medical sciences. I'd previously studied mainstream biology and psychology, so it was two years before I felt comfortable with the idea of homeopathy—an alternative medical system with its roots in the late eighteenth century and its practice based on carefully diluted and natural medicines.

Then came an epiphany of sorts: homeopathy did indeed work in the student clinic. It was indeed scientifically validated. There were no real side effects from its treatments. But it also suffered from a great shortcoming: a homeopathic remedy never held its course of healing unless the patient's case was resolved for what homeopathic practitioners know as "obstacles to cure." These are the obstacles—observed in almost every case—presented by diet, lifestyle and genetic code that impede the homeopathic medicine from having its full and lasting effect. Practitioners often seemed confused as to why a patient's recovery was only temporary and the patients often judged homeopathy not to work. This insight—that homeopathic medicines, no matter how effective in the short term weren't effective in the long term unless the practitioner addressed diet, lifestyle and constitution—led me to my passion for preventative nutrition, preventative antioxidant medicines and preventative vitamin/mineral supplementation. It was my search for the "obstacles to cure" that allowed me to grasp the idea that the actions of free radicals are the underlying cause of all disease. Ultimately, that insight led to my becoming a practitioner of what is now being called "functional medicine" as opposed to "alternative" medicine.

The shortfall of alternative medicine, as I came to see, was that it was stuck in the alternative posture, forever opposing the developments of science-based medicine. Conventional medicine, on the other hand, was stuck opposing many good ideas accepted by alternative practitioners. The medical profession has been highly effective in treating acute and life-threatening conditions and should be held in high regard for that ability. But where I saw regular medicine routinely fail was in the preventative realm and in the treatment of chronic disease. That's where natural medicine's search for the underlying causes of illness and its aim to resolve the patient of obstacles to cure can make a real difference. It was clear to me that integrating so-called alternative ideas with the discoveries of medical science was a rich field waiting to be explored.

One of mainstream medicine's main concerns has been our vulnerability to bacteria, viruses and parasites—the bad guys of the traditional medical drama, which are collectively and politely referred to as "microbes." We holistic practitioners recognize microbes as ancient agents of human misery, but we're convinced that an individual's personal level of health decides his or her reaction to infectious disease agents. Microbes have been with us for eons. Without them, we wouldn't have evolved to what we are today. In other words, it's not solely the trillions of agents themselves—the bacteria, viruses, parasites and all the other uglies—that cause disease. Our individual characteristics must play a role, or we'd all be dead from infection. Scientifically educated holistic practitioners recognize that pathogens such as viruses, bacteria and funguses are often major contributing factors in ill health, but *they are never the reason why we succumb to illness and eventually die.*

Some people get sick when exposed to a flu bug, whereas other (even unvaccinated) people show no debilitating symptoms. Granted, certain people are immune, or perhaps partially immune, as a result of a previous exposure to the organism. But others simply deal with the invader effectively, showing no symptoms of long-term consequence. These individuals clearly possess a robust immune system. Scientists acknowledge that theoretically there could be people who are totally immune to the Ebola virus, bird flu and even HIV, yet have never received protective treatment of any sort. If you are in good health when you are exposed to an "ugly," your front line defences may deal with the offending agent before your system is even breached. In other words, the level of our response to disease-causing agents depends on our genetic makeup and general health. The search for a single pathogen—a single external agent—as the cause of a particular disease has driven much of modern medical science, but finding that single pathogen is not the whole solution to treating disease.

It now appears that our health is the end result of many cumulative factors. One of these factors is toxicity. Historically, natural medicine has been much concerned with toxicity, but now even staunchly conservative scientists no longer consider the idea far-fetched. Later, we're going to have a close look at the insidious and accumulative effects of toxic substances in our environment, especially those recently introduced by humankind.

But what underlies our responses to both microbes and toxins? When it comes to this question, informed natural practitioners are geared to search for fundamental causes, an approach they share with scientists everywhere. This is the same approach that led me to the concept of the *human health threshold*.

THE HUMAN HEALTH THRESHOLD

I've practised homeopathy and functional medicine for nearly a decade now and my present practice focuses on improving the health of thousands of patients. I treat people with everything from eczema to Parkinson's disease, the common cold to cancer. Some of my special interests are digestive ailments; cardiovascular support; mood and emotional imbalances, including depression and insomnia; immune dysfunction and autoimmune diseases such as lupus, multiple sclerosis and arthritis; hormonal issues such as menopause and andropause; and autism and attention deficit disorder. I've been able to help people lose sixty or more pounds and keep it off through diet and a healthy lifestyle. Patients who've been struggling with chronic or life-threatening conditions often view the improvement in their health as something of a miracle, but I always stress that there is no miracle to natural medicine: the miracle is in the way your body works when you bring mindfulness to bear. The addition of antioxidant nutrients derived from nature simply gets your body doing the things it does best to heal itself.

My experience with my patients has brought home to me in so many ways that human health consists of an interplay of variables that include our genetics, our environment, our toxic load, our stress accumulation, our nutrition and emotional state, our exposure to microbes, our level of fitness and a plethora of other factors. Each of us has an individual ability to cope with these factors. The limit of that ability—the point at which, if we exceed it, our health fails—is our human health *threshold*.

If we imagine a thermometer that registers the sum of all these interacting factors, our health threshold is the boiling point. But the human health threshold is not a predetermined, fixed point, the health equivalent of 100 degrees Celsius; it is unique to each of us. Our capacity for managing those influences that affect our health is not a matter of simple arithmetic. Nonetheless, when we are pushed past our individual thresholds, we are no more able to remain healthy than water can prevent itself from boiling when it's heated to the boiling point. Today many of us run so dangerously close to that threshold that we increase our probability of an early decline in the functioning of our bodies. We may be living longer than the generations who came before us, but we are living longer with chronic disease and discomfort.

Let's slip the imaginary thermometer under the tongue of a person who appears to be healthy enough. He gets up in the morning, he goes to work and with sufficient caffeine he seems to be able to rise to any work crisis. This person—let's call him Will Powers—is a moderately prosperous stockbroker of forty-six whose personal health threshold is 110 degrees. Will has some poor genetic factors running in his family—early cancer *and* heart disease. These factors raise his health "temperature" to 40 degrees. You can't do what Will does for a living anywhere except in a busy city: the urban environmental burden raises his temperature another 30 degrees. You've probably guessed that Will is a type A personality and this emotional factor accounts for another 20 degrees, bringing him to 90 degrees. Okay, so he also prides himself on being no-nonsense when it comes to his food: he likes his steak and french fries. His dietary factors add 30 degrees. The result: Will's current health status is 120 degrees, well over the 110-degree threshold. He's ripe for disease at any time. The longer he stays above his threshold, the

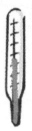

THRESHOLD
How to stay under the boiling point
You need to test your free radical levels regularly. Checking your free radical levels will soon be considered more important to maintaining your health than testing your blood cholesterol levels.

more likely he's going to develop whatever his genetic code has in store for him—probably heart disease or cancer. But if he acts fast, he could prevent the disease that's on the way.

Our health "temperature" constantly changes with our changing levels of stress, environmental burdens, and our eating and exercise habits, just as the mercury in a thermometer slides up and down in response to changing temperatures. Though Will has little awareness that he's running 10 degrees above his health threshold, he nonetheless decides he can't stand the pace another minute. He decides to drop out for a time to take a job as a deckhand on a buddy's yacht. As soon as he's on board, his daily stress drops by 15 degrees. He's eating better, too, so his diet factor improves by 20 degrees, dropping him further, to 85 degrees. Now his body can better deal with the varied health challenges—such famous infectious agents as viruses, bacteria and funguses—that come aboard the yacht as it carries adventure tourists to the Solomon and Galapagos Islands. I call this margin between Will's current health status and his health threshold a *human health buffer zone.*

But though he's enjoying the break, if he is honest with himself, Will is still hungry for the excitement of the deal. Just off the Galapagos, he receives a satellite call from his old boss who offers him a promotion to vice-president, with massive stock options as a further incentive. The stress, of course, will be even greater than before. Too bad Will hasn't had a chance to read Chapter Four on the price we pay for long-term free radical overload. His burdened health status, soon to be far in excess of his threshold, threatens once again to turn on those defective genes of his. Major bonuses and further promotions lie just ahead, but so do immune-system breakdown, chronic inflammation and eventually, cancer.

OUR JOURNEY BEGINS

The fact *behind* the threshold phenomenon is that *free radicals underlie all disease*. They are the common denominator in all the components that make up our health status, and they're the largest contributor to the burden on that health status. If traditional science-based medicine had not recently begun to integrate with natural practice, that fact might not be understood today. And if *I* hadn't followed the course I followed—from bean sprouts to biology—I might not have learned about it. This book is my best attempt, based on science and what I've found effective in my own clinical practice, to describe the dramatic relationship between antioxidants and free radicals. More than that, I hope that it will become your map on a journey to excellent health.

CHAPTER 2

THE RADICAL TRUTH

In the first chapter I introduced you to free radicals and their dedicated opponents, the antioxidants. The relationship between these two classes of molecules is a curious one and one important to our health status. As you progress from chapter to chapter, I'm going to help you make the diet and lifestyle choices that will positively influence that relationship.

If we're going to learn how to deal with free radicals, we need to know something about their background and the background of their adversaries, the antioxidants. Bad guys and their opponents are always interesting. If they indeed have a truly intimate connection to humankind, how did that connection come about? How did we come to recognize them and their numerous but almost unfathomably tiny crimes and heroic rescues? That's the subject of this chapter.

OXYGEN: AN UNRELIABLE FRIEND

Some time ago—two billion years, give or take a few hundred million—life was much simpler. Among the inhabitants of the Earth during that Paleoproterozoic or "old-first-life" era, some minuscule but plentiful organisms called anaerobes busily went about their lives, most of them in swampy fluid. Anaerobe means "without oxygen." But as living creatures, they still consumed nutrients and excreted wastes. Their waste was in fact oxygen, a gas that percolated up through the slimy sludge they inhabited. Much as we now risk suffocating ourselves with carbon dioxide emissions, these plentiful anaerobes smothered in oxygen. There was nothing willing or able to clean this new oxygen stuff up as it accumulated to the point at which the anaerobes were simply swimming in it. Eventually, many of them died. Some of them managed to survive the "oxygen catastrophe" and still exist today—in our gut, for example, where they render great service to our digestion and our immune system.

This waste oxygen saturating the previously oxygen-free atmosphere turned out to be highly reactive, chemically speaking. It readily combined with other molecules, and in due course a new type of creature evolved that could actually *use* oxygen's eager reactions as a power source—a highly efficient power source, too. The rest, as they say, is prehistory.

But oxygen has forever proven to be a bit of a two-faced friend to living things. Its tendency to lively interactions made it perfect for fueling the little energy plants called mitochondria that were floating around in almost every one of the newly evolving organisms. But the same quality caused it to make mischief when it reacted with things it shouldn't—and still does. A perfect example is the spark that leaps from a fireplace to burn down a house. Without oxygen, there can be no fire—for better *and* worse. So oxygen is already a bit of a hyperactive party atom, but some kinds of oxygen carry this to extremes. Your average well-balanced atom has a nucleus at the centre, and whizzing around the nucleus is the familiar cloud of electrons—just the right number of them. Under certain circumstances, however, atoms can lose an electron or two, and such atoms then wander around

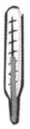 When stress is high for any prolonged period of time, the body breaks down rapidly and blood pressure can rise. High blood pressure and stress can push you over the boiling point. Free radicals are produced at alarming rates and they end up causing damage to artery linings. You're on track for a heart attack.

looking everywhere for replacement electrons attached to other atoms. These are the needful characters we call *radicals*—and sometimes *free radicals*. None of them are more reactive than the oxygen radicals.

As I said, life—that always resourceful form of matter—eventually found a way to exploit, or at least co-opt, oxygen radicals. They could be sent in to blow up bacteria that invaded a living creature. They could be used as signal runners from cell to cell within larger multicelled creatures. But oxygen radicals could never be trusted, then or now; they're just *too* radical. Living creatures have struggled to evolve ways and means of neutralizing these feckless allies since the very beginnings of life. How successful have we been? That's part of the message of this book.

THE SEEKERS

In 1954, in the depths of the Cold War, Dr. Denham Harman was studying the effects of radiation on human biological systems at the University of Berkeley in California. He was searching for viable antidotes to the sort of radiation poisoning that would result from an atomic attack.

Free radicals had been studied by chemists since the first one was discovered in 1900, and Harman understood that complex free radical reactions could result from radiation exposure. He also understood that what made radiation exposure so dangerous was that it triggered the production of the *hydroxyl* radical, the most powerful and deadly oxygen radical known—one that cannot be neutralized by the evolved defence systems of the human body. Large doses of radiation, of course, cause cancer or death, but Harman noticed that *mild* radiation poisoning produced symptoms similar to premature aging. Since low levels of radical molecules occur naturally in the human body, he wondered if the slow release of naturally occurring free radicals might be responsible for aging and for disease processes. In other words, though radiation-produced radicals were quicker, and therefore deadlier, there might be a connection between them and the free radicals produced by the day-to-day metabolism of the body.

I've mentioned that antioxidants are molecules that (as their name suggests) neutralize oxygen radicals without becoming unstable themselves. During the early years of Harman's research, certain antioxidants were already known to provide protection against radiation exposure. Harman took the next conceptual step. In 1956 he published his free radical theory of aging, which became one of the most widely accepted explanations for the aging process. Harman's theory proposed that a byproduct of oxygen metabolism in the human body—free radical molecules—can react chemically with the molecules of cells and their DNA, breaking necessary links and chains and disrupting structures and eventually bringing about the process we call aging—and ultimately death. By 1957, Harman had demonstrated that antioxidants, by neutralizing free oxygen radicals, could extend the average lifespan of laboratory mice.

Despite Harman's pioneer work, at the time most biochemists were interested in free radicals only for their important role in the manufacture of plastics. These molecules were regarded as too short-lived and too uncontrollable to play any role in serious life-and-death processes. But then, in 1961, Leonard Hayflick and Paul Moorhead, working at the Stanford University School of Medicine, determined that normal cells can divide only a limited number of times, after which cells effectively commit suicide. The number of times a cell is genetically programmed to reproduce, dubbed the "Hayflick limit," varies from species to species. In the case of human cells, the Hayflick limit is about fifty and is directly linked to the lifespan of individuals. Put bluntly, it's difficult for you and me to live on when our cells are preprogrammed to conk out after so many recycles. Here, suggested Hayflick and Moorhead, might be the truth about aging.

As work in this area progressed, it turned out that free radicals played a role in this programming. In fact, free radicals have turned out to be nature's preferred mechanism of self-destruction when a cell's time is up. The scientific name for this programmed death is "apoptosis."

In the last thirty years, free radical research has led to profound biochemical, biological and medical advances. Our knowledge of radicals has grown, and as it has grown, it has enhanced our understanding of how DNA mutates and the important role radicals play in cancer, cardiovascular disease, stroke, Alzheimer's disease, Parkinson's disease and autoimmune diseases.

Meanwhile, the study of antioxidants has also moved forward. Dr. Lester Packer, a senior scientist at Lawrence Berkeley Laboratory, was among the first to describe the role of antioxidants in the health of organisms. He proposed that antioxidants function not singly but as a *network* to balance overall free radical activity. Packer demonstrated that antioxidants synergize with one another and, even more importantly, recycle one another. In order to neutralize free radicals, antioxidants need to work like a team of firemen putting out a fire: some man the

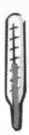

People who live to be 100 or older have higher levels of antioxidants in their bodies than less long-lived individuals.

pumper truck, some are up the ladder, some are at the hose. Some move right in close to the fire to put out the flames, where others help the victims of smoke inhalation back away from the fire. You can't get away with sending only one antioxidant—say vitamin E—into the fray: that would be like having all the firemen rush to the end of the hose, with no one left to turn on the water. As you'll learn later in this book, using single antioxidants in high doses can actually do you more harm than good.

Dr. Packer has focused, rightly, on the synergy of antioxidants. He has described five pivotal antioxidants, which he calls *network antioxidants:* alpha-lipoic acid, coenzyme Q_{10}, vitamin C, the naturally occurring forms of vitamin E, and glutathione. His conclusion: there's a synergy between these antioxidants that slows aging and prevents and treats disease.

No one disputes the value of antioxidants in diet, where nature provides them in useful combinations. Recent studies have suggested that high doses of certain antioxidants (especially taken without their necessary "network") may have marginally *increased* mortality in some studied groups. Packer's seven hundred scientific papers and seventy books on every aspect of antioxidants and health have exposed the shortcomings of those studies and maintain the importance of the network effect. The clear message that emerges from Packer's review of the literature and from his own work is that antioxidants should be taken as a balanced network and at doses specific to the individual case or condition.

A case in point. Acne often improves with a therapeutic dose of vitamin A, somewhere in the range of 10,000 IU twice daily with food depending on an individual's age and weight. However, the antioxidant vitamins C and E are also indicated for healthier skin and collagen formation and aid vitamin A in helping to get rid of the free radicals that are the cause and the result of acne formation. Cardiovascular disease, especially artherosclerosis (plaque formation), responds very well to vitamin E, but vitamin E works much better to sweep up the mess left from artery injury and plaque formation if vitamin C is also there to "recycle" its potency.

Support for the critical role of antioxidants in human health now flows in from many sources. Dr. Bruce Ames, currently project director at Children's Hospital Oakland Research Institute, is widely recognized for his pioneering research in the field of micronutrients—that is, nutrients we consume in small amounts—and antioxidant therapy. Dr. Ames has suggested that when antioxidant and micronutrient intake is low over a long period of time and damage to the cells' DNA begins to multiply, the body exercises a sort of triage system that may actually accelerate degenerative diseases and aging, eventually putting an end to the compromised organism—you—before you can pass on your DNA imperfections. This may be equally true whether you're a starving African refugee or an overfed but undernourished North American.

As a result of an intensive burst of investigation into free radicals, we now know much more about the personalities of these chemical brothers. We know that certain of these molecules—the Abels, as it were—are essential components of the body's enzymes and immune system. Others—the Cains—damage DNA and lead to cancer and other diseases.

We know now that there's a link between an excessive burden of free radicals (called oxidative stress) and aging, as when free radicals formed by excessive exposure to the sun's ultraviolet light lead to cataracts. We know that cholesterol is only one component of plaque formation, the other component being the first step: free radical damage to the arteries. (Only *then* do plaque deposits begin to form.) We know that free radical disruption of the brain may lead to Alzheimer's and Parkinson's diseases. And we know that once our body is in self-attack mode—think of autoimmune conditions such as arthritis—free radicals dominate.

This new knowledge has already made itself felt. The shelves of our local pharmacy are laden with antioxidants, and growing numbers of medical practitioners urge us to include antioxidant-packed citrus and berries in our diet and take as many as dozens of antioxidant supplements every day.

As I said in the first chapter, free radicals are directly or indirectly related to every medical condition known to us. At the molecular level, *free radical damage is the cause of all disease.* What we have yet to take on board in mainstream health circles is that what happens at the molecular level inevitably affects our overall health. I hope by the time you've finished the book, I've persuaded you of that fact.

RADICALS AND ANTIOXIDANTS UP CLOSE

When I was a kid, I saw a movie called *Fantastic Voyage,* about a submarine and its crew that were miniaturized and sent into a human body to save the patient's life. Never mind the scientific and logical problems the story presented, I'll always remember those scenes where the submarine cruised upstream through the arteries. Even today, when I think about what goes on inside the human body at the cellular and molecular level, I like to picture that submarine. I can't think of a better way to imagine free radicals and antioxidants in action, so perhaps you'll join me now on my own brief but fantastic voyage into the inner workings of a woman I'll call Rhea Gretts. Like Will Powers, she's a busy person. But unlike Will, she's uneasy about her health and much more worried about the impact of some of her bad habits. I've treated many women like Rhea in my practice. They have good instincts about what will make them healthier, and good intentions about trying to shed those last bad habits, but they've hit stumbling blocks on the way to good health.

Our journey begins as our submarine, the *Corpuscle,* is injected into Rhea's bloodstream as part of a new investigative procedure that allows patients to go about their daily lives while the medical detectives do their work.

We white-knuckled first-time investigators struggle to look calm, cling to our armrests and stare out the portholes. At the helm, the commander barks orders into a speaking tube as the *Corpuscle* tumbles through the dark surge of the heart's right atrium, the turbulence of the right ventricle, the straits of the pulmonary semilunar valve and with a final rushing roar enters the massive pulmonary artery. The blood here, depleted in oxygen, is tinted a dark blue. In the seat beside me, a young scientist states the obvious: "We're being swept into the lung. See? The blue is already turning to red as oxygen dissolves back into the blood."

We slow as we enter the smaller arteries. Outside our portholes a stream of tumbling shapes dance past us.

"The round red ones are the red blood cells," she says.

"I know." I try to smile.

"Look!" She points out the window. The artery walls are pale here and appear closer to the ship. "A plaque deposit!"

Our captain pulls back on the throttle as we slip through the narrowed passage.

"Oh dear," says my companion. "I hope this person is being careful with her diet." The artery widens again and we motor forward. The path forks, and again the walls close in. Seemingly from nowhere, a fleet of immense and ghostly spheres crowd by us and stream ahead. One slows, lingers, then extends a tentacle-like arm. I shrink from the porthole. A leukocyte apparently wants to sample us.

"Damn these white cells!" snarls our captain. "Hold on!" Our ship lurches left, evading the pseudopod, then accelerates away. An instant later we're jolted by a pulsing shriek that fills the ship.

"The smoke alarm!" shouts the skipper. "Damn! Our patient has gone out for a cigarette!" He throws a series of switches and a desperate quiet descends on us.

The young scientist whispers. "The lungs are in spasm and the alveoli are paralyzed. She's *inhaled*."

"We have to dive!" the captain warns. "We can't risk being caught by a cough."

I tighten my seatbelt, and the view outside our portholes fades to grey as we shrink down, descending from the anatomical level to the cellular level where the gross movements of the body will affect us less. A moment later the scene clears to reveal a breathtaking vista. The artery wall that had seemed so close when we were larger is now a far and glittering skyscape of individual cells. Every cell in the array looks like an immense and translucent airship. Around and between these huge shapes and on every side of us, molecules swarm.

"Damn smokers." Our captain's voice rumbles in the quiet. "Free radicals everywhere." Sure enough, we hear a hail of pings on the hull as free radicals spew from unseen reactions around us. A host of these wildly reactive molecules, indistinct except for flashing spikes and prongs, collides with the distant artery wall and cuts a swath through the helpless cells that comprise it, broken cells drifting free as a tear opens in the artery. Yet further on, the scything radicals simply disappear as if by magic.

"Now *that's* surprising," I say. "Those radicals are being absorbed harmlessly in the artery walls. There're no holes at all."

My companion nods. "There have *got* to be lots of antioxidants around here for those walls to take that sort of punishment." She squints at a drifting flock of identical molecules. "Yes! Look! Those are vitamin Es! I can tell by the shape. *Maybe* we're in the body of a smoker who's trying to eat right."

"That's a start," I admit. "Maybe she remembers to take her ACES"—which are the great antioxidants and radical killers, vitamins A, C and E, and selenium. They might be doing the job here.

The captain squeezes us through the narrow entrance to a lymph duct. Without warning, the ship lurches in a sickening arc and is dashed against the duct walls. The lights flicker.

"That damn cough again!" the captain mutters. "Hold tight!"

The *Corpuscle* is seized by a force of indescribable fury. The hull groans, the lights flicker again and go out. Darkness.

A diffuse glow outside the porthole. The captain is peering at his screens. "Yes," he says. "That cough shot us right through a lymph node and into a breast duct."

"Look at those big things over there!" My companion is pointing. "Know what they are?"

"Of course," I say. "Molecules."

She shoots me a pitying glance. "Those are estrogen hormones," she says. "They're trying to communicate instructions by docking in the duct cells, but they can't. Plastic molecules have got here first and they're mimicking the estrogen. I *hate* to see this!"

We've drifted into a spacious cavern. As the ship turns, a cluster of strange-looking cells comes into view off the starboard bow.

"Oh dear!" Her voice is tinged now with real alarm. "Those cells are multiplying out of control. That's a cancer starting." Even as she speaks, a dark shadow falls across the scene. I look up to see the great sprawl of a macrophage approaching. This is the big eater of the cellular defence army. One tentacle gropes tentatively towards us and two reach towards the multiplying cells. The *Corpuscle* draws back as the macrophage extends its pseudopods on either side of the cancer cells and with excruciating slowness engulfs them.

"I never get tired of seeing that," mutters our skipper.

The young scientist is enthusiastically explaining. "Those cancer cells are finished. The macrophage cell will dissolve them in a flood of free radicals."

"And do you think that the macrophage cell will itself be destroyed by the radicals it releases?" I ask just to see if she knows her stuff.

She shakes her head. "Not if this person is getting enough antioxidants in her diet to sweep up the aftermath." And she's right. But as the *Corpuscle* heads for the surface and the outside world, I reflect that even if that macrophage and all the rest of Rhea's white blood cells survive, all the vitamin C in the world won't keep her healthy if she doesn't stop smoking.

FREE RADICALS: RUST UNDER THE HOOD

On our excursion into Rhea's cellular realm, we got a glimpse of this fact: every cell in the body—heart cell, liver cell, blood cell—functions like a miniature chemical factory. Besides the many battles between immune system cells and bacteria, viruses and cancers, a huge number of varied and necessary chemical reactions occur inside our cells during regular metabolism. These chemical reactions break large molecules down into smaller molecules or synthesize new molecules from smaller building blocks. Other reactions transfer electrical charges from one chemical substance to another. In the course of these reactions, oxygen atoms are routinely stripped of electrons and free radicals are born at an astonishing rate. If free radicals are the cause of all disease, they must be everywhere—and so they are. Where there is life, there is the free radical—friend and foe.

The best documented formation of free radicals is those that occur when we are exposed to environmental toxins: automotive emissions, industrial pollutants, cigarette smoke, various sources of radiation (including x-rays and the sun's ultraviolet rays) and food additives, to name just a few. Study after study over recent decades has shown that lifestyle factors also contribute heavily to the formation of free radicals. Emotional stress, physical trauma, pollution, alcohol, cigarette smoke, deep-fried foods and overly strenuous exercise—these and a host of other things contribute to higher levels.

Free radicals are also formed as a not-so-obvious by-product of routine metabolism and inflammation processes. Such radicals may go largely undetected, yet they too contribute to the onslaught of oxidation that causes damage to our cells—even their destruction. If these electron-robbing, disease-causing molecules are not neutralized quickly, degenerative diseases and faster aging are the result. In many respects, the damage done by free radicals in the human body is similar to the rusting of a machine. Rusting is, after all, the reaction of the iron with those very oxygen radicals that "rust" our bodies. Here's a homey example: we've all noticed that apples turn brown after their flesh is exposed to air. That too is oxidation. To slow down these oxidation processes, we apply protective paint to the iron and squeeze lemon juice on the apple. Paint temporarily keeps the oxygen at bay; lemon juice contains vitamin C and limonoids, both of which are powerful antioxidants.

ANTIOXIDANTS: NATURE'S ARMOUR

We've seen how life is continually exposed to oxidative stress from inside and outside the body, and how living cells and entire organisms have developed defence mechanisms—various types of ingenious "antioxidant armour"—to protect them against free radicals. Essentially, antioxidants work by neutralizing free radicals, donating their own electrons to the hungry radicals while simultaneously maintaining their own stability as molecules. It wouldn't do if antioxidants neutralized free radicals and were radicalized themselves in the process.

Our trillions of cells are abundantly equipped with these free radical defence mechanisms. But when we're on the receiving end of an onslaught by chemicals, viruses, bacteria or mutant cancer cells, our defences are often overwhelmed. If we're to prevent this cellular struggle from erupting as an actual disease, our cells require extra help. When it comes to our personal health, we don't have another ten thousand—or a hundred thousand—years to evolve that help. That's why we can benefit from eating certain foods and taking certain antioxidant supplements that help our cells do their jobs without sustaining significant damage. Of course *some* damage happens as we age, just that little bit, day by day, but it's the small and acceptable amount of aging that we must think of as inevitable.

There it is then—one of the most important messages in this book: *Sufficient antioxidant protection helps prevent ill health by stopping the chain reactions of free radical damage that underlie all disease.*

THE BALANCING ACT

Radicals cause great harm, yet paradoxically, we cannot exist without them. At the molecular level, every time we fight a cold, try to remember something or feel sexually aroused, we're putting free radicals to use. Our immune cells produce copious numbers of the free radicals nitric oxide and superoxide, which are indispensable to such good deeds as opening blood vessels and "poisoning" invasive viruses and bacteria. Our immune system employs certain free radicals to *kill* cancer cells before the cancer grows, as we imagined on our submarine adventure.

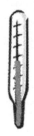 Vitamin D is an essential vitamin and antioxidant important to our overall health and prevention of cancer. There is no better way to get it than responsible exposure to the sun. However, when you spend too much time in the sun, the free radicals that accumulate from the sun radiation can actually *cause* skin cancer.

In fact, many cancer drugs work by temporarily *increasing* the production of free radicals in the body. Oncologists also use focused radiation to generate powerful free radical activity and so *destroy* a cancer tumour. Yet free radicals in great numbers—those generated by our immune systems, say, or by too much *un*focused radiation—can eventually *cause* diseases such as cancer. What are we to do with this contradictory evidence?

The governing principle behind all biological processes is *homeostasis,* a Greek-derived word meaning balance. We'll have cause to refer to balance again and again throughout this book. The body must maintain an internal free radical balance. Unfortunately, for reasons we've already glimpsed, most of us are very imbalanced indeed, with far too many free radicals loose in our systems. So new is this knowledge, few people—including doctors—yet know what a free radical *balance* really means or how it might be achieved.

In the chapters that follow, we'll explore the phenomenon more deeply. And then we'll turn to real-world no-guess ways by which you can determine the current levels of free radicals in your body and establish that life-enhancing (and life-prolonging) balance.

ARE FREE RADICALS REALLY THE ROOT OF ALL DISEASE?

A skeptical lay researcher once bet a bottle of good red wine that he could stump me on my contention that free radicals are involved in all disease. He proceeded to present me with the following scenarios.

Skeptical Investigator: A nurse is pricked by an HIV-contaminated needle and eventually dies of AIDS. How does she die of free radicals?

Bryce Wylde: The role that free radicals play in the case of HIV and AIDS is variable throughout the disease. From initial infection to full-blown AIDS to death—every step includes free radical bombardment at the cellular level. As an acquired immune-deficiency virus, HIV attacks the body by using a process of illusion so that the body can't recognize it as a foreign invader. Paradoxically, in the first stages, the immune system doesn't initiate *enough* free radicals in order to kill off the virus. When a person develops full-blown AIDS, death doesn't come from the AIDS virus itself, but from the onslaught of free radical-related injury caused by every other disease that the person is now unable to fight off. This can include conditions otherwise as benign as the common cold.

S.I.: How about someone sickened by the malaria parasite?

B.W.: The malaria parasite sparks the body's immune system response into employing the necessary free radicals. This attack on the parasite inevitably damages many other nearby tissues and organs. As one example, free radical overload can cause kidney failure and ultimate death if the person doesn't receive immediate help.

S.I.: Okay, take heart failure from a purely mechanical clogging. What do free radicals have to do with a 103-year-old man dying of heart failure?

B.W.: No matter the person's age, a heart attack or heart failure or heart disease *always* involves free radicals. As blood is the carrier of free radicals as well as their neutralizers, the antioxidants, the linings of the arteries are often the site of free radical "thunderstorms" that cause everything from plaque accumulation to heart attacks. Interestingly, it's not the cholesterol itself that causes the plaque accumulation. The culprit is the original injury to the artery lining caused by a cascade of free radicals that *then* causes plaque to deposit at the site of injury.

S.I.: What about a woman who dies of an aortic aneurysm?

B.W.: In nearly every case of aortic dissection or aortic aneurysm, free radicals are the initial cause of the compromised vasculature. Years of free radical damage eat away at and weaken the walls of the artery or outpouch them enough that you may bleed outright into your body or brain.

S.I.: Okay, so take a fellow bitten by a cobra. He dies. Surely . . . ?

B.W.: Death from a snakebite is a case of toxic shock governed by free radical overload. Nearly every toxin found in cobra venom initiates a tremendous amount of free radical damage and interrupts blood-clotting platelet-aggregating factor. At the molecular level, this causes major, irreversible damage by instigating "reperfusion injury." Your organs melt from intense free radical onslaught as if you were exposed to nuclear radiation and you end up bleeding to death from the inside out. If the fellow is lucky enough to survive, it would be because a heroic dose of antivenom stopped the free radical cascade. He'd also need some significant doses of antioxidants to clean up the rest of the free radical inflammation that may continue for years after the actual encounter with the snake.

S.I.: A depressed person commits suicide . . .

B.W.: Free radicals are almost always involved in depression. As one example, some forms of psychoses and mental disillusionment can result from improper "methylation." Methylation defect is a deficiency of specific antioxidants, including folic acid, the antioxidant B vitamins and vitamin C, especially in cases of schizophrenia. Free radicals are notorious for their attack on the nerve fibres in cases of depression caused by chronic stress, dementia and Alzheimer's disease.

S.I.: (*flipping through his notes*) An air traveller dies of deep vein thrombosis. How could that be caused by free radicals?

B.W.: In this situation, a person may occasionally die of end-state organ necrosis or infection, both of which are free radical induced. But generally, the cause of death is acute. The most obvious example is thrown emboli, carried in the blood into the brain or heart or lung tissue, which causes immediate restriction of blood flow. The real question is what causes the emboli in the first place. The most frequent causes are oxidation of cholesterol, homocysteine or some other pro-inflammatory agent that instigated free radical damage at the arterial level. These and other free radical events can all lead to emboli, and emboli cause deep vein thromboses.

S.I.: All right, how about the case of a two-year-old child who dies of polio?

B.W.: Polio cannot be prevented or treated with antioxidants, but polio *is* a viral disease just like the common cold except that polio puts out a free radical toxin that destroys anterior horn cells in the spinal canal. Polio, as with many other deadly viruses, is also the cause in this case of a flurry of other free radical attacks by the body's own immune system on the virus—all too often such an intense attack that the body can rarely ever regain balance. In the end, the nervous system is severely impaired or the poor child dies.

S.I.: And if the child dies instead of cancer of the retina?

B.W.: Any cancer, neoplasm or cell mutation is initiated by an attack on the genetic code.

S.I.: An attack by . . . ?

B.W.: By free radical molecules. Often the result is a battle for control between *free radicals* and antioxidants. Due to an imbalance of cell regulation, natural killer-cell activity springs into full action. An entire host of other DNA and immune-related oxidative stress ensues.

S.I.: Forget cancer then. A fifty-year-old dies of amyotrophic lateral sclerosis—Lou Gehrig's disease. Now what will your radicals and antioxidants do?

B.W.: Free radicals are the cause of the nerve death due to an autoimmune attack sequence. This causes loss of function, and can end up causing the untimely demise. No doubt you see no way antioxidants could help here. But they might surprise you. Strong antioxidants such as phosphatidylserine and *N*-acetylcysteine don't offer a cure, but may help slow the progression of the disease by slowing down the deterioration of the nervous system.

S.I.: What if an automobile accident victim dies of shock? That's something we can all understand. It's basic. It's down to earth.

B.W.: In this case, the body shuts down—and fast—due to a process known as cellular "autolysing." In hypoxia— lack of oxygen from asphyxiation or extreme cold—cells begin releasing a huge number of deadly enzymes that destroy all other surrounding cells and injure tissues by initiating a cascade of free radicals. It's as if we all at once "rust" thousands of times faster than we do via the natural aging process.

S.I.: Okay, okay. But allow me to pose my *coup de grâce.* A stabbing victim dies of blood loss.

B.W.: Clearly a tragedy, but obviously this situation does not qualify as disease, and of course I acknowledge the point at which disease and trauma separate.

CHAPTER 3

THE CAUSES OF OUR FREE RADICAL BURDEN

The program I outline in this book is going to help you create a healthy balance between the antioxidants in your body and "oxidative stress." I've already mentioned some causes of oxidative stress, but in this chapter we're going to have a closer look. You'll already be familiar with many of these causes—they're clearly harmful—but what might be less obvious to you, as it is to people when they first come to see me at my practice, is how the actions of free radicals link these factors to our health.

A woman I'll call Maria recently came to my clinic with symptoms of both chronic fatigue syndrome *and* fibromyalgia, including debilitating fatigue and persistent muscle pain. But she didn't have the typical history—she had never had the Epstein Barr virus. Her blood on a general screening showed nothing remarkable, but when I tested her free radical levels they were very high.

Next I tested hair and urine samples for the presence of toxins, and found high levels of arsenic and mercury. I started Maria on alpha-lipoic acid, a strong antioxidant, immune regulator and heavy metal mover. I raised and lowered the dose over the course of treatment depending on her urine analysis results. I also pre-scribed three months of oral chelation therapy to bind and draw the toxins out of her system. After six months, her free radical levels had dropped to normal ranges and the heavy metal levels in her hair and urine had dropped to almost nil. Maria said she was pain-free and that she had not been so energetic for at least ten years. In my practice, I find that both chronic fatigue immune dysfunction syndrome (CFIDS) and fibromyalgia are both on the rise not because of the virus that has been linked to them but because of our toxic diets and environment.

TOXINS

A few decades ago, you rarely heard the word "toxin." If some-thing could poison you, you called it "poison." Everyone knew what poisons were. They were the products labelled with a skull and crossbones: the caustic lye in the garage, the bleach in the laundry room, the bottle of iodine in the medicine cabinet.

Today, toxin is a word on everyone's lips, perhaps literally. Late-night infomercials—which of course none of us watch—deliver urgent, low-budget warnings about toxins, then offer us the miracle of detoxification. We're familiar with detoxification too—"detox" as the health-store clerks cozily call it—every celebrity seems to sign up for it. It's a painless process, this detox-ification, normally requiring little more than following the prod-uct directions on a bottle and eating, say, beets for a month. A tremendous value at $399.99, plus local taxes where applicable.

Most of us at least nod in recognition when toxins are men-tioned, but, if my practice is anything to go by, we don't give them much effective thought otherwise. We've all splashed our-selves a few times with a corrosive cleaner while cleaning the toilet. We may share our region with a nuclear reactor. We've drunk municipal tap water all our lives. Somehow we're still here to read this book.

The topic of toxins can seem like new-age vagary elevated to news status by a hungry media; bowel flushes and lymph cleanses sure seem like the brain hatchlings of tree-hugging vegans and fringe health fanatics. In the face of a flood of information, what are we supposed to do, put on a radiation suit when someone walks into the office eating a non-organic apple?

Scientists once thought that the womb protected developing babies from toxic pollution. But a new study of umbilical cord blood from newborns found an extensive array of industrial chemicals, pesticides and other pollutants. In 2004 researchers at the Environmental Working Group in Washington, D.C., tested cord blood from ten newborns for the presence of 413 chemicals, including a diverse range of pesticides, flame retar-dants and stain- and grease-proof coatings. The newborns aver-aged 200 contaminants, and the study identified 209 pollutants that had never before even been detected in cord blood.

Since the Second World War, an estimated 85,000 synthetic chemicals have been registered in the United States alone. Toxico-logical screening data are available for just 7 per cent of these chemicals. This means that tests can detect only one in fourteen chemicals. If 200 trace chemicals were found in a newborn, we might in theory be looking at as many as 2,800 synthetic chemi-cals in one small body.

I'll discuss below the dangers of the plastics that deliver our food. But producing that food employs an array of pesticides, insecticides and herbicides to kill the insects and weeds that harm the crops. These obvious toxins run off from fields and enter the water table; we've all heard about their effects on our collective health. Sometimes we may think about it when we pass the little organic produce counter at the supermarket, where a small number of worried souls (including myself) prefer to buy their food. You too may choose to buy there. But as I contemplate the vast stocks of non-organic fresh produce elsewhere in the store, I'm compelled to wonder: if it weren't for pesticides, would over 300 million North Americans even have access to these healthful, nutrient-rich fruits and vegetables?

We try to improve our standard of living, and the new adhesives, carpets and building materials outgas volatile organic compounds. We sand away the pre-1960 paint, and so release lead into our homes. We tear down old ceilings in schools and offices, and invisible threads of asbestos insulation float out to lodge in lungs and produce mesothelioma, a usually incurable cancer.

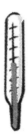

Diabetes shortens your life span in part because it depletes antioxidants and creates high levels of free radicals. Diabetes will keep you close to your boiling point, but antioxidants can decrease your risk of complication and increase your longevity.

We demand our dentist remove the amalgam from our teeth, and we're told we'll release a flood of mercury into our bodies. We attempt to eat more healthily by upping our fruits and vegetables, and in doing so are exposed to levels of pesticides strong enough to cause neurological disease if we are so predisposed. And if or when we finally succumb to the toxic burden and go to see our doctor, he or she prescribes us a medication that is likely to increase our total level of free radicals. Is there no escape?

For our purposes, the important fact is this: a growing body of scientific evidence supports the idea that toxins are toxic because they increase our free radical burden. If we know what we're dealing with, we can act to use antioxidants and changes in the way we live and eat to reduce that burden. Let's start by looking at some broad categories of familiarly "toxic" substances.

Plastics

They're everywhere and we love them. We wear them, slip our feet into them, see through them. We sit on them, eat on them, eat *from* them, eat *with* them, walk on them, drive around in them, watch them and play with them. The synthetic polymer, a critical component of the chemical industry, has in many respects *become* the very substance of our material lives.

The first "plastic" was invented about 1910 by Leo Baekeland, who called it Bakelite. Since then, industrial chemists have churned out a polysyllabic catalog of plastics: polymethylmethacrylate (Plexiglas), polyesters, polyethylene, polyvinyl chloride (PVC or vinyl), polyhexamethylene adipamide (the original nylon polymer), polytetraperfluoroethylene (Teflon), polyurethane and a host of others. But these new substances have been in existence for just a few generations; only now are we beginning to understand the impact they're having on our health. And so dependent are we on plastics, even if it were proven tomorrow that they were directly linked to cancer, it might take decades—if ever—to find an alternative that would be accepted and mainstreamed. In 1945, a year after Baekeland died, annual plastic production in the United States had reached some 400,000 tons. In 1979, the annual volume of plastic manufactured overtook that of steel, the classic symbol of the Industrial Revolution. Today there are over 50,000,000 tons of plastic produced annually in North America.

Ana Soto is a medical doctor and a professor at Tufts Medical School. Her main research interest for the last twenty-eight years has been breast cancer. In 1989, with Dr. Carlos Sonnenschein, she discovered that certain types of plastic—bisphenol A and epoxy resins—emit chemicals that mimic the female hormone estradiol and can cause breast cells to multiply in cancerous fashion. Even more recent research, from the biological sciences department of the University of Missouri, suggests that infants and children are unable to flush bisphenol A from their system. Formula from plastic bottles and plastic-lined cans exposes children to worrisome amounts of the synthetic estrogen. This plastic exposure (especially in our youngsters) during the past half-century may account for the observed swift increase in the lifetime risk of breast cancer. In the 1940s, a woman's lifetime risk of breast cancer in the United States was 1 in 22. Today, the risk is 1 in 8. Breast cancer is the leading cause of death in women aged 34 to 54. This increase cannot be attributed to genetics alone; the increased risk of breast cancer and other cancers has paralleled the proliferation of synthetic chemicals. Researchers are now implicating the outgassing from plastics in other hormone-sensitive cancers. Common household items such as toys, carpets and computers are being linked to other conditions, such as asthma and migraines.

As government agencies have come to recognize the dangers of plastics, some regulation has been put in place. You can look at Appendix B to see how plastics are categorized according to their chemical types. Not all plastic containers are labelled, but several deserve special mention.

PVC (category #3) is used in food packaging, including plastic trays for boxed cookies or chocolates, candy bar wrappers and bottles. Cling wraps, including the kind used commercially to wrap meats, cheeses and other foods, are often made of PVC. Traces of toxic chemicals—especially the phthalates used to soften PVC—can leach into our food, especially fatty foods at higher temperatures. (Never microwave your food in plastic, nor cover it with plastic wrap while heating or freezing it; this enhances the contamination.) We are all exposed to these chemicals every day, but we *can* lessen our children's exposure. PVC is commonly used in teethers and soft squeeze toys for young children, in beach balls, bath toys, dolls and other products such as knapsacks, raincoats and umbrellas. Again, scientists are increasingly aware of the dangers of phthalates and concern is rising for children who play with these soft PVC toys.

A recent study in *Environmental Health Perspectives* concluded that some styrene compounds leaching from polystyrene food containers are also able to mimic estrogen and may therefore disrupt normal hormonal functioning. Worryingly, styrene is also considered a possible human carcinogen by the World Health Organization's International Agency for Research on Cancer. To get a sense of just how extensively we're exposed, the next time you go shopping, take a look inside your (plastic) grocery bags and ask yourself this: Every week, when I arrive home with the groceries, do I also want to deliberately swallow a pill that could cause cancer? If not, it's high time to make some hard decisions about using alternatives to plastics.

Ironically, many plastics regarded as "green" or "healthy"— those used in Nalgene bottles, the big water bottles used for water coolers, Brita pitchers, Avent and other baby bottles, most plastics with recycling number #7 on the bottom, the lining of tin canned foods, and the various dental "sealants"—contain bisphenol A, the potential estrogen-mimicking agent and hormone disruptor. Some studies have suggested that bisphenol A may have a negative impact

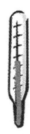

Flossing your teeth can add a year to your life by reducing inflammation of your gums, and as a result your free radical levels! Good oral hygiene helps keep you under your threshold.

on our health, even at the parts-per-trillion level—the equivalent of one drop of chemical in a lake. Such a finding is alarming since most chemicals are marketed as having a safe "threshold" for consumption. The plastics industry acknowledges that leaching can take place at parts-per-billion levels—leaching of most chemicals found in plastic is more likely to take place through heating or when the container is scuffed, scratched, old and worn—but disputes the claim that parts-per-trillion levels could be harmful. As a practitioner of homeopathy, which often employs medicines in ultradilute form, I know that parts-per-trillion can aid in recovery. So I'm inclined to believe that other substances, similarly diluted, could cause harm. Health Canada announced further testing on bisphenol A—one of two hundred chemicals—in 2007.

What is the link between plastics and free radicals? When an error in cell division results in the "daughter" cells having the wrong number of chromosomes, that error is called "aneuploidy." In some cases there is a missing chromosome; in others cases an extra one. A great deal is known about the effects of aneuploidy, but less is understood about its causes. Many scientists suspect that the underlying cause of aneuploidy is free radicals, which attack the genetic code, and thereby replace good code with faulty code. When this happens early in conception—and it often does—it is called "meiotic" aneuploidy and results in the spontaneous miscarriage of the fetus. The human body is usually ingenious in its ability to detect and deal with mutation. But babies who survive to birth after aneuploidy are likely to have birth defects, including Down's syndrome: meiotic aneuploidy causes 10 to 20 per cent of birth defects in people.

Another type of aneuploidy is associated with almost all solid-tumour cancers.

The free radicals generated by the plastic toxin bisphenol A have been implicated in both these types of genetic mutations.

I don't want to overwhelm you all at once with all the chemicals and other harmful substances that daily life brings us in contact with. Our chemical industries work day and night to produce stuff we want and—more often than not—believe we need. The book you're holding, for example. The paper mill that made the paper digested trees to make a pulp and separated the fibres from the impurities, then bleached, dewatered, pressed and rolled the pulp while emitting plenty of nitrogen oxides, sulphur dioxide, dioxins and greenhouse gases. If the pulp mill didn't do that, you couldn't be reading this now. And you wouldn't be reading anything else either. That's the modern dilemma.

Shampoo, shaving cream, lip gloss, hand soap, dish detergents, laundry detergents, moisturizing creams, perfumes, air fresheners, cosmetics and deodorants. In our heart of hearts, we know these useful little additions to our daily lives start out as nasty raw materials—we just don't like to think about it.* Dyes and pigments, rubber, the fabrics that make up our clothing, the paint on our houses, the tube of glue in the kitchen drawer—we know they started out in places with chimneys belching sulphur oxides, nitrogen oxides, volatile organic compounds, particulate matter, carbon monoxide, sulphuric acid, carbon dioxide and dioxins. We know—but we don't want to know.

In fact, I don't want to bog you down here with worry on your path to better health, so for more info please consult Appendix B, where, along with the plastics list, I provide information on automotive toxins; dioxins and furans; pesticides; heavy metals, including mercury, arsenic and lead; and the impact of radiation, including the sun's rays, radon gas and mobile telephone radiation.

---

* There's a fine online database at http://www.ewg.org/reports/skindeep/ ?key=nosign that enables users to search the safety rating of a product.

But I do want to spend some time on certain important areas that burden our systems with excess free radicals every day.

Food Additives

Of course we want food that is fresh and hasn't spoiled so that it doesn't poison us. We want food to look fresh too, even if it isn't. We want it to smell good, feel good and taste good. The food industry, to whom added preservatives have always been important, continues to respond to our desires with an array of enhancers. In Appendix C, I list a few you can chew on the next time you open a package of chips, cookies or almost anything eaten from a package. I refer to them as "unknown" and "sneaky" ingredients because only limited literature supports their negative side effects, but manufacturers know that we're beginning to look for them because users increasingly attribute side effects to them. To keep us guessing, manufacturers often resort to derivatives with slightly different names and acronyms.

When most food came from farms, shopping was in fact easier and food more nutritious. Now, factory-made foods have made chemical additives a significant part of our diet. Most people may not be able to pronounce the names of many of these chemicals, but they still want to know what the chemicals do and which ones are safe, which are poorly tested and which may be possible causes of their health complaints. Serious studies have thrown the safety of many food additives into doubt, or condemned them altogether. A simple rule about additives is to avoid those found in the charts in Appendix C. Not only are they among the most questionable additives, but they are also used primarily in foods of low nutritional value.

I know that it can be hard to take warnings about additives too seriously. After all, they appear in famous products, brightly lit in the aisles of supermarkets. Can they really be so bad? Yes, they can. The Additive Cemetery is filled with sweeteners, preservatives and colourants once accepted as safe and now banned altogether.

What about those "natural" additives, sugar and salt? They seem so harmless, these brother crystals, and processed food manufacturers wouldn't dream of selling you a product without one of them—usually both of them. But sugar in excess causes inflammation and cellular damage; salt imbalances electrolytes and can cause high blood pressure and may in fact be a major contributor to our present-day epidemic of hypertension. Together they may pose the greatest risk of all because we consume so much of them.

Like industrial toxins, food additives are so pervasive it's difficult to avoid them entirely. That's why I want you to understand that they exert their destructive effects—when they do—through the mechanism of free radical action. Choice examples are the additives glutamate and its derivative monosodium glutamate (MSG). Glutamate, when added to products above the natural levels found in food, can cause excess free radicals in our cellular mitochondria that cause deterioration of cell membrane function; that damage seems to be a contributing cause of oxidative neuron death in neurodegenerative disorders such as Parkinson's and Huntington's diseases. MSG, the sodium salt of glutamate, at dose levels above 4 mg/g of body weight has been shown to induce oxidative stress and free radical accumulation in liver cells. Many of us have come to know the after effects of MSG as "Chinese restaurant syndrome"—a nasty response to too much MSG that can range from headache to stomach upset and diarrhea.

Prescription Drugs

As a society we generally believe that maintaining health is as simple as occasional restoration through a prescription written by our doctor for a drug produced by the pharmaceutical industry.

We don't normally think of prescription drugs as toxic since our doctor has told us to take them to combat a malady. We believe that we can often achieve a quick and easy fix for something that is the result of a lifetime of poor choices.

All drugs have side effects; we're familiar with that notion. But a side effect is actually a nice way of saying a *primary* and unwanted effect that a prescription medication may have on your body. The simple fact is, *all* drugs cause toxicity, and this is especially likely when they are used for reasons other than those intended. The abuse of over-the-counter drugs is especially widespread. Acetaminophen, for example, the active ingredient in Tylenol, has recently been shown to have far more toxic effects on the body then previously believed, even after a few doses. Scientific studies show that acetaminophen induces profound elevation of free radicals and oxidative stress and reduces the levels of our own natural antioxidants.

It would be too much like high school chemistry class to lead you through the broad range of pharmacopoeia and biochemical side effects of major prescription drugs. But allow me to partially summarize by drawing on the work of Dr. Ray D. Strand, whose recent book *Death by Prescription: The Shocking Truth Behind an Overmedicated Nation* addresses this issue. He writes that the leading drug problem today is not the use of illegal drugs, but the use of *legal* prescription drugs. Strand argues that prescription drugs are five times more likely to kill you than an automobile accident or AIDS. The fourth leading cause of death in the United States is *properly* prescribed and administered medication. Add improperly prescribed medication, and prescription drugs become the third leading cause of death. Strand cites over two million hospital admissions and 180,000 deaths each year in the United States alone due to adverse drug reactions.

There is a time and place for all modalities of medicine—including pharmaceutical drugs that are properly prescribed. But when you decide to accept a precription from your doctor, you need to know that taking the drug will increase the free radical burden in your body. The pressure of a drug-induced free radical burden affects the liver. Every drug you ingest (including caffeine and alcohol) ties up liver enzymes and puts a strain on the body's supply of antioxidants. In a healthy liver, antioxidants transform harmful free radicals into harmless water-soluble substances that the body gets rid of through urine, feces, sweat and even breath. Over the long term, any prescription medication causes the liver to become hindered and sluggish, and raises the amount of free radicals in the body. By virtue of the pharmaceutical drugs we are pushing through our systems, we raise our free radical load enormously.

IMS Health is a pharmaceutical information and consulting company with a presence in over a hundred countries worldwide— just about every major pharmaceutical and biotech company in the world is a client. IMS recently reported that global spending on prescription drugs in 2005 topped US$600 billion. To put this into perspective, the estimated economy of the *entire world* in 2006 was at US$65 trillion. That means that for every hundred dollars in circulation around the globe, approximately one dollar is being spent on prescription medication. For example, Pfizer's cholesterol pill, Lipitor, is the best-selling drug in the world, with annual sales of US$12.9 billion, more than twice as much as its closest competitors: Plavix, a blood thinner from Bristol-Myers Squibb; Nexium, a heartburn pill from AstraZeneca; and Advair, the asthma inhaler from GlaxoSmithKline.

Armed with the knowledge that certain drugs increase your free radical load, what are you to do? The simple answer is to read on and then follow the instructions in the action plan of the book: you'll cover all your bases no matter what prescription drugs you're taking. But I've got some immediate and simple answers for people taking the most common prescription drugs on the market for your heart. If you're taking Lipitor for elevated cholesterol, take the antioxidant coenzyme Q10 (CoQ_{10}). Lipitor is among the "HMG-CoA reductase" inhibitors that create a deficiency of CoQ10 in all of your cells and result in the breakdown of your tissues causing kidney damage and sore achy muscles. Consider taking 100 mg of CoQ10 twice daily with food.

If you're taking Plavix, you'll be happy to know that there is no known free radical side effect from it. It may actually *protect* against free radical accumulation. However, you might want to research nattokinase as a potential and effective natural alternative to Plavix, since the drug has been known to cause abnormal liver function and clotting disorders.

Lastly, perhaps you've been put on Norvasc for high blood pressure. (This drug represents about US$5 billion in annual sales.) Norvasc is a calcium channel blocker and may also protect you against certain free radicals that may be damaging your artery linings. But it may cause free radical damage in the kidney. If you are taking this drug, I would strongly recommend that you consider 100 mg of alpha-lipoic acid daily as a part of your antioxidant supplement routine.

METABOLISM

We say that our bodies "burn" food to generate energy. What we mean is that our bodies' cells combine oxygen with food molecules for this purpose: it's important to remind ourselves that this fundamental metabolic process produces oxidative stress. Research is now confirming what common sense would suggest: too much or too little of certain foods will affect the numbers of volatile radical by-products we produce.

If you eat more than your body needs to generate energy, it forces you to metabolize fuel that your body doesn't need, which it stores as fat. This metabolic process causes the accumulation of excess free radicals. Heart disease at the level of the artery doesn't start with deposits of plaque; it starts well before that, with free radical injury to the lining of the artery. It's *after* the free radical injury to the lining of the artery that your body initiates the healing response by depositing the plaque.

And, of course, damaging, free radical-generating substances—pollutants and micro-organisms—can enter our bodies *with* our food. But beyond this indirect role in sickness, our diet's greatest contribution to our health lies in choosing what we eat to balance our free radical burden. In the chapter on nutrition, we'll look specifically at how to employ the powerful antioxidant tool that diet can become.

EXERCISE

If our diet is the sum of what we take in—the fuel of our metabolism—then exercise represents part of the other side of the metabolic process: our energy output. Since, like any burning of fuel, the metabolic process is an oxidative process, it's not surprising that too little or too much exercise will affect our free radical levels.

Too Little Exercise

We all know that not getting enough exercise is bad for our health. Heart disease—along with artery lining dysfunction, plaque formation, the storage of toxins and fat and poor circulation—are all proven consequences of inactivity. It's our predominantly sedentary lifestyle—not to mention overconsumption—that prompts our doctors to warn us so frequently to *start* exercising (or keep up the good work) if we want to remain free of cardiovascular disease. The ultimate consequence of too little activity is free radical strain on the liver. Down at the molecular level, our cells succumb to "metabolic syndrome"—later known to patients as a combination of diabetes, heart disease, hypertension and obesity.

Too Much Exercise

You may consider "hero" athletes such as cyclist Lance Armstrong to be the epitome of health, and for the most part they are. But where many of these athletes fail is in their antioxidant protection routines. I can't prove it, but I suspect Armstrong contracted cancer in part because of the excessive free radical-producing exercise routines that were necessary to win the Tour de France seven times in a row. Tests have shown that Armstrong has a high aerobic threshold (the oxygen-carrying capacity in his blood) and can maintain a higher tempo or cadence (often 120 rpm) in a lower bicycle gear than his competitors. This style is in direct contrast to previous champions, who used a high gear and brute strength to win. But the high-cadence pedalling style, which allows the leg muscles to recover faster, and so allows the cyclist to sustain effort for longer periods of time, transfers the stress to the heart, which is at higher risk of free radical damage.

Lactic acid is responsible for the feeling we get when a muscle is exhausted—often a cramp under the rib cage from running beyond our ability. The most unusual aspect of Armstrong's physiology is his exceptionally large heart and lung capacity and his ability to maintain low lactate levels. He consequently feels less fatigue from extreme exertion.

But it's actually right there where a substantial amount of free radical damage may be done. Lactic acid often acts in the body as a delayed "stop" signal. There comes a point at which, depending on our level of athleticism, our muscles, lungs and heart are not supposed to endure further oxidation and free radical damage, and free radical damage to DNA and body tissues begins to accelerate. In my opinion, Lance Armstrong had some cancer code ravelled deep within his DNA that said, "Slow down, Lance. If free radicals turn me on, you'll get testicular cancer." Lance couldn't hear those genes, of course.

STRESS

Stress is a collective, scientific-sounding term for our more unpleasant emotions. Some people still find it a bit surprising to see the connection between our "mind"—our subjective thinking and feeling—and changes in body chemistry that scientists can actually measure. In fact, the link between mind and body has been intensely investigated in recent decades and some remarkable findings have emerged.

Here's an example. You've probably heard everywhere, for example, how omega-3 fatty acids and other so-called essential fatty acids (EFAs) are *essential* to humans and yet cannot be synthesized by the body. They must be obtained through our diet and our diets are often strikingly deficient in them. That's why we're starting to see signs in supermarkets advertising products such as eggs and dairy with added "omega-3." You might assume that the big benefit of the essential fatty acids is to your heart or arteries. But a host of laboratory and population studies suggest that the biggest benefit of essential fatty acids is that they are important to our *mental and emotional health*. Countries where diets are deficient in these fatty acids show a higher incidence of mental illness. A lack of essential fatty acids has also been implicated in Alzheimer's disease and Huntington's disease. Other studies have demonstrated that the addition of EFAs to diets can relieve such conditions as depression, bipolar disorder and even schizophrenia.

So it should come as no surprise that stress—obviously a feature of our mental lives—affects our physical selves at every level.

You and I may never have been the sort of child who would put a kitten in a harmless headlock just to watch it squirm in desperation. But anyone can understand the experience well enough: being threatened while

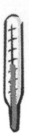

The risk of cancer and heart disease is considerably lower in people who consume 5 to 7 servings of antioxidant-rich fruit and vegetables daily.

being forcibly constrained is terribly stressful. I mention the kitten because—like it or not—researchers investigating stress have subjected animals to something similar in order to analyze the chemical outcome of this so-called immobilization-stress state. They have found it to be associated with increased free radical production, decreased antioxidant enzyme levels, increased oxidized lipids in tissues (which has been linked to heart disease) and oxidized lipids in brain tissue—linked in some studies to degenerative brain diseases. This free radical activity has in turn been found in human studies to be clearly associated with impaired cognitive function. Major stress for a single eight-hour period increases oxidative stress and free radical attack on the brain, with accompanying decline in memory and cognitive function. Antioxidant nutrients have been shown to mitigate these effects when administered before or after the stress-induced circumstances.

The chemical specifics of stress go something like this. We're unexpectedly faced with the prospect of losing our job. With the speed of light, a chemical cascade begins. Our nerves fire off from the various awareness centres to the hypothalamus, deep inside the brain. There, a hormone known as CRH is released directly into a connecting pathway to our pituitary gland. The pituitary now secretes its own hormone known as ACTH straight into our main bloodstream. ACTH acts on our adrenal glands (little pyramid-shaped structures that sit on top of our kidneys) causing them to release cortisol and adrenalin. These hormones arouse our body to meet the presenting challenge, and they do so with such intensity that the cells of our organs begin working overtime. Of course free radicals—the natural result of accelerated body processes—begin to appear. When this happens too often, the free radicals cannot be neutralized and become truly harmful.

Acute stress, with its knee-jerk reactions, happens too quickly to register consciously, but we soon experience dramatic physical changes that we interpret as "stress": the dry mouth, the sweaty palms, the racing heart, the shallow breathing, the burst of physical energy. If the stressful event is exciting and not just awful, our brain releases the feel-good chemicals serotonin and dopamine. We may or may not exhibit behaviour that may or may not qualify as temporary insanity. Then a suborgan of our brains—the amygdala—may step in to play a delayed role as regulator. Eventually our serotonin and dopamine levels decline, perhaps leaving us depressed and emotionally frazzled. At last, when we've had time to debrief ourselves, input from the sensory regions of our brains is edited and filed away as a learned experience. However, this debriefing mechanism is always a little late to stop a flood of free radicals.

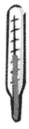 Moderate exercise helps you stay under your boiling point. But too much exercise can have a bad effect on your overall health. If you work out intensely for more than 14 hours a week—without adding balancing antioxidants to your diet—you'll cause unhealthy free radical elevation.

Chronic long-term stress caused by lack of sleep, deadlines, always rushing, always being on the go, is clearly a factor in aging. When someone is subject to this sort of stress, we can almost see them age before our eyes: their expression changes, their posture changes, their voice changes.

Now it's time to recall the kitten in the headlock. The great dilemma of stress in modern humans is that our brain chemistry is outdated. We simply haven't had time to fully evolve into *Homo technocraticus*. Our reactions evolved under conditions of physical dangers hundreds of thousands of years ago in order to help us defend ourselves when we were attacked by sabre-toothed tigers. But when these primitive responses to stress appear in the face of dangers that call for no physical response, they become an added burden to our health—we're like stressed-out kittens held immobile by our lifestyle—and this burden pushes us towards our personal health threshold. Today, ringing telephones, dinging emails, looming deadlines and abstract responsibilities threaten to overwhelm us and elicit the prehistoric chemical cascade. Unfortunately (and, well, fortunately), we encounter telephones and computers far more often than our distant ancestors encountered sabre-toothed tigers. The effects of cortisol and the other stress hormones, when they flow through the blood for too long and in too concentrated a form, are highly undesirable and lead to uncontrolled weight gain and, of course, elevated levels of free radicals.

Elevated levels of oxidative stress may not be the only consequence of stress. Loss of our protective antioxidant factors is just as destructive. In studies at the Department of Neurology, Medical College of Wisconsin, researchers placed subjects under controlled stress by having them study for tests and depriving them of sleep. The results were measurably lower levels of protective antioxidants in the blood, leaving the subjects vulnerable to free radical attack. It's easy to extrapolate from this the effects of sustained stress. Studies on psychological effects of stress in the work force suggest that the higher the employee's stress, tension and anxiety, the higher the damage done by free radicals to their DNA.

We should hardly be surprised that stressful events trigger molecular events inside our bodies. Our modern view is generally that the mind cannot be separated from the body and, for more than half a century, science has been bent on demonstrating this. Researchers have induced such subjective experiences as fear, calm, anger and psychological stress in laboratory environments and traced the biochemical cascade of brain chemistry that is implicated in these feelings. The findings are conclusive: We are endowed with an intricately woven neural net that connects the psyche to visceral health. The brain—the seat of the subjective mind—can be shown to have a direct effect on such "chemical" systems as immunity and genetic expression.

Just as you can't separate mind from body, you can't separate mind from the immune system. The immune system responds automatically to viruses and bacteria and other foreign molecules just as the brain responds automatically to stress. And these two response systems respond to each other, working constantly together to maintain an internal balance.

Our nerves link the brain to every organ and tissue in our body and to those very organs responsible for stress responses. Challenging or threatening situations arouse the brain's stress response and this process releases hormones that regulate the immune system. But if you've already reached your health threshold, a variety of molecular, cellular and behavioural responses may go so far as to initiate self-attack. Under ideal circumstances, any time your body has been invaded by a foreign organism, your immune responses would attempt to counteract the looming threat. But when your individual threshold has been exceeded, the body's resources are simply spread too thin to come to your aid, and the body breaks down.

Contemporary science is just beginning to understand the many ways in which the brain and the immune system are connected, how they help to regulate and balance each other and how they can malfunction and produce chronic disease. When my patients report a point since which they've "never been well"—a bout of pneumonia, say—I explain that this episode wasn't what caused them to develop their later disease. It was simply the one that brought their system to the "boiling point." Now, treatment becomes, in part, a matter of *mind*: if we do nothing more than establish a positive thought process, we reduce the burden on our threshold and begin the healing process.

The "mind" doesn't just affect the "body." It works the other way, too. A series of recent studies suggest that if we have an infection or an inflammatory condition, or any ailment for that matter, and free radicals begin to circulate in our blood at higher than desirable levels, the result may be a clinical depression. Your biology becomes your psychology.

You'll remember our friend Will Powers from Chapter One, the broker with the borderline health threshold. Will has long had a recurrent cold sore that crops up every time he loses sleep, works too hard or get stressed out, which is pretty often since he went back to work as a broker. These cold sores are a type of herpes virus and a perfect example of the *psychoneuroimmuno-modulatory* phenomenon. Will picked the virus up from a nice girl when he was eighteen and, although his first cold sore healed after a while, the virus has stayed dormant at the dorsal root of his spinal cord, only to peek out again whenever his immune system's attention is diverted. This is especially likely when Will exceeds his health threshold, which—yep—he's doing again. When his stress-triggered cortisol levels have remained high long enough, such that his immune system is sufficiently depressed, his first-line defence is effectively sidetracked and there's the sore on the same spot on his lip.

This interwoven mind-body-immune relationship of nerves, hormones and organs also regulates our food intake and reproductive behaviour. Prolonged exposure to stress can lead to such unhealthy and unappealing developments as infertility and belly fat. Will Powers hasn't been too troubled about his sperm count recently, but he *has* noticed that his abdominal muscles are things he has to dig his fingers in to find these days.

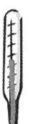

Vegetarians, on average, live longer than non-vegetarians, and have higher levels of antioxidants in their bodies. Eating too much red meat pushes you to the boiling point.

EVERYDAY LIFE

If you think that with careful living you can avoid all sources of oxidative stress, think again. Mitochondrial energy creation—the process within our cells that powers our bodies—creates free radical accumulation, just as exhaust is the consequence of an internal combustion engine. In fact, simply living and breathing day to day is a primary source of free radical accumulation in the body. That's why we creatures have evolved an internal cellular antioxidant capacity—our antioxidant armour—to neutralize free radicals. But our internal capacity to neutralize this metabolic, free radical exhaust is not enough. Day-to-day metabolism seems to cause the creation of more damaging free radicals than there are antioxidants to clean them up. Our bodies need help, and if they don't get it, we pay the price in ill health.

CHAPTER 4

THE PRICE WE PAY FOR CARRYING OUR FREE RADICAL BURDEN

Before we embark on the antioxidant prescription I am going to propose, let's look more closely at some of the most important consequences of a radical-antioxidant imbalance.

CANCER

You remember Leonard Hayflick, whom I mentioned in Chapter Two? It was Hayflick who in 1961 made the melancholy announcement that the maximum number of times a human cell can divide is about fifty-two.

Science has since confirmed Hayflick's findings. This limit has been noted in all human cell types that have evolved for specific functions—mature, fully differentiated cells—and in the cells of other organisms too. The limit varies from cell type to cell type, and from organism to organism. But in our case, the number to remember is fifty-two. Every time the cell divides, the telomere—which is the region at the end of the chromosomes that acts as a sort of safety mechanism to prevent over-replication—gets shorter, like the fuse on a bomb. When there is no more telomere left, self-destruction is initiated. This cell death is called apoptosis and is executed in such a way as to safely dispose of cell corpses and other cellular remnants. Between fifty billion and seventy billion cells die each day due to apoptosis in the average human adult. In a year, this amounts to the proliferation and subsequent destruction of a mass of cells equal to your body weight.

There are at least two types of cells that are immune to the Hayflick limit. One type is the stem cell, an immature cell whose job throughout the course of our lives it is to regenerate new cells as the old cells hit their Hayflick limit.

The other immortal cell is the cancer cell. In fact, it is now believed that the Hayflick limit evolved principally *to help prevent the development of cancer.* But cancer cells have found the way around the limit and are able to prevent the destruction of their telomeres.

And now the punchline. The mechanism most likely to cause cells to ignore the telomere signal is *free radical activity.* An ionizing ray of radiation from the sun, for example, may zip right past your top layer of skin and cause a flurry of free radical formation that in turn breaks the DNA gene that encodes the "stop" signal on a skin cell. So the cell keeps on dividing and years later, a melanoma develops, the deadliest of skin cancers. But if you had an antioxidant in the vicinity that neutralized that free radical and prevented it from damaging the DNA, then the outcome would be different. It's almost that simple. An extra bit of vitamin A floating by that day may have saved your life.

Let's look quickly at two typical studies that reinforce the link we now see between cancer and free radical damage to our DNA.

An article in the August 2003 edition of *Cancer Research* ("Products of Oxidative DNA Damage and Repair as Possible Biomarkers of Susceptibility to Lung Cancer") described how, in some lung cancers, increased levels of oxidative DNA damage is associated with tumour formation and progression. The implication of this research is that it may be possible through blood analysis to assess the types and concentrations of DNA damage in cancer patients. The resulting "fingerprint" may allow better diagnosis and a better assessment of the patient's response to treatment. In fact, these damaged-DNA fingerprints may permit us to detect the onset of cancer in otherwise "healthy" people well before it reaches the point of no return.

In the same year, an article in *The Breast Journal* ("Volatile Markers of Breast Cancer in the Breath") reported a correlation between breast cancer and free radicals and described an effective test for detecting free radicals on the breath, a test that may permit screening for breast cancer.

The first of these studies tells us something important about how the cancer begins and progresses through genetic mutations induced by free radicals. The second study links testable free radical levels—even on the breath—to breast cancer. In both cases, free radicals are at work mutating genes. We can make a reasonable assumption that these radicals can be combatted with antioxidants found in food and supplements. Clearly, understanding the cancer-triggering mutations free radicals can give rise to—and the genetic predisposition of the individual—will be crucial to the deployment of targeted antioxidants.

STROKES

A stroke is another too-common human affliction that can be laid at the doorstep of the free radical. A stroke occurs when blood flow is cut off or restricted to a particular region of the brain. It could be caused by a blood clot, or by a piece of debris that breaks off from plaque and blocks the artery delivering oxygenated blood to the brain. Whatever the cause, the results are devastating. Free radicals almost certainly play a role in the long-term cause of the plaque formation, but when a stroke does happen, much of the physical damage to the brain does not immediately occur when it is deprived of blood and oxygen. Most of the damage actually occurs *following* the stroke, when the blood flow is restored. This is called reperfusion injury. When the "old" blood in the brain mixes with the "new" oxygenated blood, there is a thunderstorm of events that cause free radicals to accumulate at alarming rates and injure tissue some distance away from the original event. They may also attack nearby tissue, resulting in permanent brain damage. That's why it is so important to treat any stroke with strong antioxidants. It's critical to consult with your cardiologist about intravenous antioxidant treatment and chelation therapy following a stroke. This option is extremely helpful in recovery, but it has only just recently been considered viable. Be patient with your specialist if he or she isn't yet implementing it. But whether it's as sudden and catastrophic as a stroke or as chronic as the degeneration of Alzheimer's disease or dementia, losing our minds is the effect of uncontrolled free radical accumulation.

HEART DISEASE

Free radicals are involved in both the onset and the progression of heart disease in several different ways. When we think of heart disease, we're most likely to think of the acute scenario of chest pain or heart attack. Heart disease, like mental decline, is too often accepted as a natural consequence of aging. It doesn't have to be. Granted, along with aging comes some degree of "hardening" of the arteries. This is to be expected, just as you'd expect the wrinkles and sags we'll talk about in the next section, "Aging." But true heart *disease* starts well before the first symptoms are ever felt.

At the beginning of this process, free radicals attack the lining of the inside of an artery. If the interior lining of the artery is repeatedly injured, the body's natural response is to deposit cholesterol plaque at the site of the injury, much like putting little Band-Aids on superficial wounds. If there is too much low-density lipoprotein (LDL)—also known as "bad" cholesterol—in the system as a result of a poor diet or other unbalanced variables, the deposition of oxidized LDL will continue long after the repair is accomplished. The body, in other words, may not know when to stop applying the Band-Aids. The result will be ever-growing plaque deposits.

In recent years, Dr. Makoto Suzuki, cardiologist, geriatrician and former director of the Department of Community Medicine at the University of the Ryukyus in Okinawa, Japan, established the Okinawan Centenarian Project to study the extraordinary longevity of the people of Okinawa. Dr. Suzuki's study had found that one of the *best* common denominators for living longer appears to be blood levels of high-density lipoprotein (HDL)—

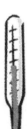

Once or twice a year improve your health status by detoxifying your body, safely, and you'll help maintain your human health threshold at healthy levels.

the *good* cholesterol. When cholesterol levels are unhealthy, the process of plaque deposit may take many years, but when an artery is finally clogged with plaque, the result may be a sudden loss of blood and oxygen to the heart—a heart attack.

Yet here's something that might surprise you. Most of the damage to heart muscle inflicted by a heart attack is caused by a burst of free radicals *after* the blood flow is resumed, very similar to the stroke scenario. Those of us unfortunate enough to experience a stroke but fortunate enough to be taking antioxidants will always fare better in recovery. One free radical in particular, nitric oxide, may play a central role in this destruction (and one antioxidant, vitamin E, may play a key role in cleaning up the damage). Yet nitric oxide is essential for normal blood circulation. Clearly, it's a balance we require. And the same holds true for the commonly misunderstood cholesterol; it's simply not all bad, as we've just learned. Cholesterol is crucial to the function of our hormones, our immune system and to the artery-repair system.

AGING

Just because aging is not in itself a disease doesn't mean it isn't a consequence of free radical activity. We can think of aging as the accumulation of random damage to the building blocks of life—especially to the DNA and to certain proteins, carbohydrates and fats. This damage begins early and eventually exceeds the body's self-repair capabilities. It gradually impairs the functioning of cells, tissues, organs and organ systems, thereby increasing vulnerability to disease and giving rise to the characteristic manifestations of aging: loss of muscle and bone mass, a decline in reaction time, compromised hearing and vision, graying of the hair, reduced elasticity of the skin—the list goes on and on.

Reduced elasticity of the skin is in fact one of the most observable consequences of this natural and inevitable aging process. Topical creams loaded with false-hope antioxidants that are supposed to slow down the aging of the skin—few actually do—serve to fuel the anti-aging industry. But it is true that free radicals damage a skin protein called elastin that holds the cells of the skin together and gives it flexibility and strength. Sooner or later this elastin skin will sag and appear wrinkled and discoloured. Without free radical attack on elastin, we might be indistinguishable at eighty-five from our high school graduation pictures.

Aging—that is, remaining alive over time—by definition exposes us to more free radical activity, and so makes us more susceptible to afflictions such as heart disease, Alzheimer's disease, stroke and cancer. But in my view, these age-related conditions are superimposed on the actual aging process, not identical to it. Science may some day eliminate today's leading killers of older individuals, but different maladies will take their place, and every single one of them will have a free radical connection. This aging process guarantees that one crucial body component or another—the heart, for example—will eventually experience a catastrophic failure. It is an inescapable biological reality that once the engine of life switches on, the body begins to sow the seeds of its own destruction.

FREE RADICALS AND OUR GENES

At the heart of each cell in our body—and indeed most living things—are strands of deoxyribonucleic acid (DNA), whose component genes are the unique blueprints for who we are. Although the code contained in our genes may be unique to each of us, the order in which the genes are arranged in the vast DNA molecule is more or less consistent for any one species. All the information contained in a species' DNA is called its *genome*.

We know that each of us is born with a unique genetic code, a predetermined tendency to certain types of physical and mental functioning, coded for and expressed by our genes. As scientific knowledge advances, we know that this genetic code has a great deal to say about how quickly we age and how long we will live. Although the evidence is still coming in, it appears that each of us has a biological clock that is ticking away, an alarm set to go off at a particular time, but a time that depends in part on how well we treat ourselves. When that alarm finally does go off, it signals our bodies to age quickly and then to die. Naturally, we're looking for the snooze button.

The recent decoding of the nearly forty thousand genes of the human genome has opened up an entirely new spectrum of knowledge, one that offers tremendous potential for improving our health and well-being. As we've seen, one of the outcomes of this effort is that virtually all of the most pervasive, disabling and deadly degenerative diseases of our time—including heart disease, adult-onset diabetes, cancer and senile dementia—are now believed to develop from *an interaction between free radicals and our genes*.

Science is not yet able to directly alter our genetic heritage, but evidence is rapidly accumulating that our daily choices of the food we eat, the water we drink, the rest and sleep we get and the emotional responses we sustain can modify the *expression* of our unique code—the *expression* of our genes at a molecular level— for better or worse.

Here's an example. Scientists now believe that certain sequences of our DNA code—single nucleotide polymorphisms (SNPs, pronounced *snips*)—which may vary between individuals as the result of mutations, are turned on or off depending on the amount of free radical damage that occurs in the immediate vicinity of the cell's genetic vault. Certain SNPs, turned on, can code for certain diseases. Free radicals have the potential to actually destroy our DNA sequences and cause mutation within this code for life. If the code is interrupted, our cells receive disturbed information that can lead to diseases such as cancer. This means that specific damage done to us by free radicals, whether from the sun's UV radiation or that hot dog we eat while watching the baseball game,* has influenced the genes our parents donated to

---

* I would never eat a hot dog at a game or anywhere else.

us at conception, genes that were themselves altered by free radicals in the distant past.

Thus choice plays a significant role in our health. I think we should seriously reconsider the idea that we can do nothing about the cards we've been dealt. At the very least we can play those cards well. Staying healthy enough to keep living relies to some significant extent on protecting our genetic material from free radical damage. What this confirms is that discoveries at the molecular level suggest that some of the most important challenges to our health are our toxic environment, our toxic diets, our toxic lifestyles and our toxic states of mind. These are things our ancestors didn't have to worry about nearly as much.

A BENEFICIAL EFFECT: THE ANTIOXIDANT GENES

We living creatures are not without our defences. For a little more than a decade now, study after study has demonstrated that exposure of human and animal cells to free radicals results in adaptive changes in gene expression. These changes afford the cell protection against future insult. This change in gene expression, originating from a special section of genetic code, the *antioxidant response element* (ARE), demonstrates the cell's ability at the DNA level to deal with and detoxify reactive chemicals, and so withstand oxidative stress.

Here's an example. In 1997, Wyeth Wasserman and William Fahl at the McArdle Laboratory for Cancer Research, University of Wisconsin, found that human cells exposed to cancer-causing agents, including free radicals, turned on the ARE section of genetic code. Once these antioxidant responders were turned on, they could protect the cell against cancer-causing substances and excess free radicals by increasing the number of protective enzymes in the body, such as glutathione, a powerful antioxidant that we all have inside us—although often not in sufficient quantities. It goes without saying that if we skimp on the nutrients, antioxidants and good food we need to resupply this protective function, it won't work.

Early in 2007, at the University of Pennsylvania, scientists used a novel computational tool to identify a set of AREs that had been altered by SNPs (those *snips* again—mutated versions of genes). This tool may help identify high-risk individuals with a lowered ability to fend off free radicals. These are the very people holistic practitioners—and hopefully all doctors—will want to help.

These and other studies contribute to the remarkable discovery that has flowed from the mapping of the genome—that the job of specific genes in our DNA is to respond to free radicals. As free radical molecules turn our genes on or off or even deform them, our cells respond by activating numerous "antioxidant" genes that work together to make a coordinated response to this oxidant stress. As part of that response, our cells then produce antioxidants such as glutathione. All of these genetic response systems have evolved together to reduce the stress caused by the free radical molecules to which we're exposed. And as we'll see, we could—and should—help boost this response by ingesting additional antioxidants such as vitamin E, vitamin C, the carotenoids and selenium as part of our diet and a supplement program.

CHAPTER 5

TESTING FOR FREE RADICALS AND ANTIOXIDANTS

We've looked at how our bodies host a life-and-death struggle between free radical and antioxidant molecules, and we've seen how that battle can turn against us if the forces of free radicals grow too numerous. To act effectively to redress the balance, we need to know which forces are in play and in what numbers. That's where testing—both in your doctor's office and with testing kits that I have developed that you can use at home—comes in.

Most of us have been tested for something—to see if our sore throat is actually strep throat, for instance, or to see if our blood cholesterol levels are too high.

But our main interest in this chapter will be testing not for diseases but for the *underlying causes of disease*—the imbalance between free radicals and antioxidants.

BIOMARKERS: OUR BODIES SPEAK

A "biomarker" is a substance in our bodies or other observable change that indicates an underlying state of health or disease— the presence of antibodies that suggest a present or recent infection, or sugar in the urine, indicating the possibility of diabetes. In some cases, a biomarker may point to a disease before the disease itself appears. Familiar examples are blood lipid levels— cholesterol and triglycerides—used by doctors to assess the risk of future heart disease.

If free radical activity is at the root of all disease, it's hardly surprising that free radical activity reveals itself in a wide variety of biomarkers. Conversely, if an antioxidant improves specific biomarkers, that antioxidant may also improve the quality of life— and longevity—of individuals. For practitioners of natural medicine, the biomarkers of greatest interest are those that suggest *susceptibility* to a disease. Our bodies, like our cars, have warning lights. If, when your oil warning light flashed, your first impulse was to open the hood and disconnect the annoying thing and then chug on down the

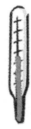

Drinking from plastic can shove your system towards its boiling point and increase the risk of cancer. Drink from glass, not plastic.

highway, the result would be a disaster—for the car. Biomarkers can be the flashing signs of compromised body systems. We must know how to read these signs.

FIRST, TAKE A GOOD LOOK AT YOURSELF

Our bodies offer an array of biomarkers that require no lab tests at all; they're observable physical signs of free radical stress that may signal a risk of potential illnesses requiring antioxidant treatment.

Hair, skin and nails play a particularly telltale role because they are affected over time by your state of health—influenced by your blood antioxidant and free radical levels—and then of course they stay around long enough to tell a story.

In each of the visible biomarkers I list below, I suggest a possible cause related to excessive free radical activity and suggest a counterbalancing antioxidant supplement. (We'll look at these supplements in more detail in Chapter Ten, "Your Personal Antioxidant Supplement Plan.")

Hair

If your hair has lost its shine, free radicals from the environment are attacking the hair protein and its natural oils. Although this is not dangerous, it is an indication that you are low on essential fatty acids. You should certainly be supplementing your diet with essential fatty acids such as fish oil.

Are you greying prematurely? This may suggest free radical attack on the pigment of your hair follicles. Take 500 mg of para amino benzoic acid twice daily and cut down on refined carbohydrates.

Is your hair is falling out? Free radicals may be attacking your thyroid. Here is where a doctor's help is necessary. Ask your doctor to test your blood for the hypersensitive form of thyrotropin (TSH), thyroxine (free T4) and triiodothyronine (free T3). Depending on the outcome of your test, you may want to start taking the antioxidant set of B vitamins (as a 50 mg complex taken twice daily with food) and the amino acid tyrosine (750 mg twice daily on an empty stomach).

Nails

Some people's fingernails show lots of white spots. Free radicals may be using up excess zinc in their immune system and causing them to be zinc deficient. If you don't have reason to believe that the white marks came by way of injury, supplement your diet with zinc citrate (10 mg a day taken with food).

If you have vertical ridges (called "Beau's lines") in your nails, your digestive enzymes—especially hydrochloric acid—may be low or you're taking too high a dose of antacid medicine. Enzyme imbalance can cause free radical buildup. Later in the chapter, we'll look at easy ways to have your digestive enzymes checked.

If your nails break easily, free radicals may be attacking your protein. Take the antioxidant amino acids glutathione (1,000 mg twice daily on an empty stomach) and NAC (500 mg twice daily on an empty stomach) and try the mineral silica in liquid form (5 mg once daily).

Skin

Warts are caused by a virus that also causes free radicals to bombard your immune system. Take a combination of vitamin A (10,000 IU a day) and beta-carotene (20,000 IU a day) with food.

If you have dry hands, you'll be interested to know that inflammation caused by frequent weather changes can cause free radical accumulation. Use lots of hand cream, wear gloves in the winter and increase your fish intake—especially deep-water fish such as fresh or canned wild Alaskan salmon, sardines, farmed rainbow trout, albacore tuna, Atlantic mackerel, black cod or farmed arctic char. These fish are among the healthiest you can eat; they are relatively clean and free of chemicals and heavy metals.

Rosacea is a rash affecting the face and chest. Often food sensitivities can cause immune responses and free radical attack in the vessels of your face and chest. When your rosacea is caused by this, vitamin B_2, or riboflavin, at up to 5 mg twice daily, ideally as part of a B-complex, will possibly clear this condition up.

If you find that cuts heal slowly, it's a good guess that free radicals are beating up your immune system. You're probably low on vitamin C and zinc. A supplement of about 500 mg of ester-ified vitamin C, with a therapeutic dose of 10 mg of zinc citrate daily with food, will improve your healing.

Easy bruising indicates a deficiency of bioflavonoid antioxi-dants such as those supplied in berries, cherries and grapes. Tak-ing extra vitamin C can remedy this and certainly do no harm.

If you've developed dark brown elbows, you need B-complex vitamins.

Excessive stretch marks may be a sign that you're deficient in vitamin A. I might suggest that you try a combination of vitamin A (10,000 IU a day) and beta-carotene (20,000 IU a day) with food.

Spontaneous nosebleeds suggest your blood vessels have high levels of free radicals, either from repeated injury or perhaps due to fragile capillaries. Either way, increase your antioxidant levels with 500 mg of vitamin C and bioflavonoids fruits such as berries, cherries and grapes.

Eyes

Dark circles under your eyes could be genetic, but the antioxidant methylsulfonylmethane (MSM), when applied topically, may help. You may also need iron and B_{12}. Ask your doctor to check your blood for signs of anemia, and consult with him or her about iron dosages.

Poor night vision is a sign that your eyes are being hit hard by free radicals caused by sunlight and aging. You'll need optimal levels of vitamin A and beta-carotene at the dosages I mentioned above in the section "Skin."

If the whites of your eyes are turning yellow, your liver may not be functioning well and your free radical levels are likely very high. Time to do a simple cleanse or perhaps even the sort of structured detoxification I'll describe later. Support your liver function using the body's strongest antioxidant, glutathione.

Even though glutathione isn't easily absorbed in pill form, I would nonetheless recommend a dose of 1,000 mg twice daily on an empty stomach. It wouldn't hurt to add some dandelion and milk thistle either. Both should be taken as herbal tinctures (liquid extracts) in standardized form. Ask your health-care provider for a personalized dosage and recommended length of treatment.

Mouth

Cracks at the corners of the mouth (angular cheilitis) can signify free radical attack on the metabolic system called methylation, which can indicate heart disease in the making, perhaps caused by candida. Take a 50 mg vitamin B complex that includes folic acid and B_{12}, and have your doctor look at your iron and B_{12} blood levels at your next checkup.

Mouth ulcers are often a sign that inflammatory free radicals are causing protein tissue destruction. Use the antioxidant power of amino acids L-glutamine and L-lysine (each at 500 mg twice daily on an empty stomach).

If you're experiencing a diminishment of taste or smell, free radicals may be building up due to allergies and the constant release of histamine. Take extra zinc in order to help other antioxidants clear the inflammation.

Do your gums bleed frequently? Perhaps you just don't floss enough. On the other hand, free radicals may be at the root of a chronic infection. Take the remarkable antioxidant coenzyme Q_{10} (more on that in Chapter Ten), and don't forget to take more vitamin C.

Inflamed gums are also helped by the antioxidant power of vitamin C. Take it to "bowel tolerance," a concept I'll explain a little later in this chapter in the section "The Vitamin C Test."

Elsewhere

Inflexibility of fingers could be the result of free radical attack causing arthritis. The antioxidant MSM at 1,000 mg twice daily will help, along with vitamin B_6 at 100 mg per day.

If your body temperature is chronically elevated or depressed, this could be your thyroid acting up, a sign that your immune system is being attacked by free radicals. It may respond to an increase in your intake of antioxidant vitamin A.

A deep diagonal line across the earlobe has long been recognized as a signal of potential heart problems. Protect yourself from cardiovascular disease by taking your antioxidant powerhouses, vitamins A, C and E, and selenium—the "ACES" of antioxidant therapy. Add CoQ_{10} to this mix and you'll be well protected. More about recommended dosages in Chapter Ten.

This list could be a lot longer, but I hope the message is still clear: excessive free radical presence in our bodies reveals itself in many ways before it results in serious disease. If we only take the trouble to observe our own biomarkers and respond with appropriate antioxidant measures, we can redress the balance. Let's look now beyond these more obvious signs to tests that you can perform at home.

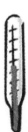

Coffee, red wine and chocolate can be good for you! Adding these in moderation to an already excellent diet can actually keep you from boiling over as they all add to your antioxidant protection.

With recent advances in medical technology, we no longer have to wait until we can see visual markers. We can act to restore the balance before we can see the signs of actual damage by accurately testing our bodies for free radical levels using blood and urine samples. Armed with this knowledge, we can modify our diets and lifestyles to minimize the damage caused by free radicals, as I'll advise later in this book.

AT-HOME TESTING

In Appendix D, I survey some pretty exotic tests that can only be conducted by skilled technicians in fully equipped labs. After reading this book, you may be persuaded that this sort of testing for free radical levels is a valuable tool in the prevention of cancer, Alzheimer's disease, arthritis, cardiovascular disease and many other diseases, and you may be convinced that current research strongly and increasingly favours antioxidant therapy. Yet you may find going to your doctor's office to explain that you want this kind of testing to be awkward, even daunting—especially if you're confronted by a condescending attitude.

For nearly a decade I have been running blood and urine antioxidant analysis for my patients at my on-site clinic laboratory as a routine part of checkups. Eventually patients began asking how they could perform regular checkups on their own at home between their visits with me. So we began five years of development work on a take-home version of the tests and today are able to offer a personal antioxidant test kit so that you can monitor your antioxidant health status at home.

The kit includes separate tests to determine your free radical levels (using malondialdehyde); to measure your vitamin C demands, which gives a good picture of your antioxidant protective status (using dichloroindophenol in reverse titration); and to check for your stress levels (using potassium chromate and silver nitrate and studying sodium overspill). I'll explain more about why I chose to concentrate on these areas in the individual test sections below.

Rather than measuring all the individual antioxidant nutrients in the body to get an idea of your total antioxidant level, which would be prohibitively costly and inconvenient, my test kit provides a simple way to ensure that you have sufficient antioxidant status. The tests are non-invasive. You simply place a sample of your urine (collected in the privacy of your bathroom from the first flow of the day) in each of the three test tubes and wait less than five minutes, then compare the result with a colour chart provided in the kit. The kit comes with an educational guide that helps you interpret the results and gives you information on how to improve your antioxidant status for optimum health. If you are able to make changes in your diet, exercise and other health habits, you don't have to guess as to the effectiveness of those changes or wait for a doctor's appointment: a retest using the kit will measure the impact on your antioxidant status.

(Bryce Wylde's Antioxidant Test Kit is now available to the public and can be purchased online at www.drwylde.com. An order form is included at the back of this book, which contains an introductory offer for those who have read *The Antioxidant Prescription*.)*

Measuring Cell Damage

We know that, in the process of free radical production in the body, certain chemical by-products arise. A substance called 8-OHdG (8-hydroxydeoxyguanosine) is the actual biomarker that points to free radical damage to your DNA. Blood testing for this substance is the most accurate form of testing free radical levels overall because it measures free radical damage to your DNA. But the test is very expensive (often more than $600), and it requires a visit to the doctor's office, specialized equipment and complicated laboratory techniques in a highly controlled environment. Another chemical by-product that arises in the process of free radical production in the body is malondialde-

---

* Results and information are for personal use only, and are not intended to diagnose, cure or treat specific diseases or conditions. This screening test was developed by HGW Inc. and its performance characteristics were also determined by HGW Inc. It has not been cleared or approved by the U.S. Food and Drug Administration or by Health Canada. For more information on the scientific basis of these tests, please see Appendix D.

hyde, or MDA for short. Levels of MDA correlate well to levels of 8-OHdG, and, as discussed, you can test for MDA at home.

In special cases, people such as AIDS patients or certain patients on chemotherapy may discover themselves to have a free radical level that is too *low*. Remember that balance is the key. *Low* free radical levels may represent an *under*active immune system response. In such cases, taking more of the wrong type of antioxidants may actually *worsen* the condition. (I have patients who never thought they'd hear me say that.) If you find your levels to be consistently high using the home analysis, you may want to invest in blood evaluation work.

If *no* free radical activity is detected, I recommend you take *no* antioxidants and would prescribe instead immune-stimulating herbs and supplements until the results indicate ideal levels.

The Vitamin C Test

Vitamin C is a powerful and famous antioxidant. Humans are among a small group of mammals unable to manufacture their own vitamin C and must acquire it through their diet. We also cannot store vitamin C in our bodies. Until the mid-1970s, it was thought that any amount of vitamin C greater than about 60 mg a day—the higher levels, for instance, contained in supplements—was excreted. But a growing number of natural health-care practitioners and some scientists were persuaded that taking megadoses of the old antiscurvy vitamin did more than prevent scurvy. Evidence emerged that vitamin C could help people avoid common colds and flu and generally improve the condition of the immune system, skin, hair and nails, among other things. New research has estimated the dosage necessary for optimal health to be 200 to 500 mg per day, not 2,000.

But some people can benefit from a much higher intake because they simply metabolize vitamin C faster than average.

The urine test I recommend measures what you take in, then use, and the by-product that comes out. If nothing shows up on the way out, that result suggests that you have used up all the vitamin C in your system and you may require more. The protocol would be to up your dose, test again, see that in fact you are ingesting ideal amounts and continue on at that same dose.

I recommend that vitamin C-deficient patients take the vitamin to "bowel tolerance"; that is, enough vitamin C to make your stool soft (not to the point of diarrhea though), starting with, on average, 1,200 mg of buffered vitamin C twice daily and going up by 600 mg a day until you notice the change in stool. Once you've observed the change, reduce the current dose by 600 mg and continue on that dose. This method is of course much less accurate than the urine test.

The Stress Tests

As we've learned, biomarkers are late-onset red flags that show up *after* there has been an initial insult to the body but before disease has fully taken hold. Waiting to observe changes in biomarkers is often a "test" too late. In the same way, checking blood pressure or blood cortisol for evidence of stress also comes too late. Why would we want to wait for the serious signs of stress to appear? Thanks to the rapidly evolving science of biological testing, you can now test for your current stress levels a lot earlier.

Stress is a highly subjective experience. The familiar physiological reaction known as "fight or flight"—run for your life or fight for your life—is integral to our survival, but the internal chemical reactions that mediate fight or flight can be triggered by something as ordinary as spilling your milk or something as extreme as being attacked on a battlefield. It depends on how you're wired. We *do* know that if you experience a fight-or-flight response too often, it leads to free radical accumulation and disease.

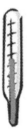

Is cancer inevitable? No! Free radical–induced cell defects can be fought with antioxidants. If our cells don't get a regular supply of antioxidants, they can be forced beyond their threshold and can proliferate into benign or malignant tumours.

In human evolutionary terms, the stress reaction was a necessary part of everyday life. Predators had to be fled from or fought. Unfortunately, this reaction can be evoked these days by being stuck in traffic as you are heading to pick up the kids from their after-school programs while you are on the cell phone with your boss and trying to swallow that fast food your doctor says you must stop eating because of your high blood pressure—and then suddenly remembering that you forgot to pick up the dry cleaning that you need for your meeting tomorrow, and that if you don't get the kids soon, you're going to be late for the evening appointment you made.

Stress—a major contributor to free radical accumulation—is the number one silent-killer, the epidemic of the new millennium. In the same way that it's best to assess your heart's current function by checking your blood pressure, the best way to assess your physiological stress is to check your adrenal gland function. When you're stressed out, your adrenal glands work overtime and stress-related chemicals flood your system, causing high blood pressure, sleeplessness, immune dysfunction, anxiety and a high cortisol hormone level that leads to weight gain. If this chemical imbalance goes on for too long, the adrenals eventually fail to produce the necessary hormones and you begin to experience burnout, depression, hair loss, salt cravings, low blood sugar, impaired liver function, chronic fatigue syndrome or a variety of autoimmune disorders.

Spikes in chemicals from stress aren't detected using the standard blood tests, and most medical doctors, if they test for, say, blood cortisol, are looking for diseases that are not closely related to stress. A natural health-care practitioner, however, will relate cortisol, catecholamines and DHEA (more on all these later) to your adrenal aptitude, which has a direct correlation to stress and the way it affects you.

An assessment of your adrenal gland function can help a clinician identify factors that may be strongly contributing to other disorders or setting the stage for serious health problems in the future. We can then significantly alleviate disease symptoms associated with high or low levels of cortisol, catecholamines and DHEA—particularly those that are age related—with a therapeutic program of exercise, diet, stress reduction and supplementation. Since both excesses and deficiencies of DHEA and cortisol have been implicated in various stress-induced illnesses, preventative and therapeutic approaches should emphasize the critical importance of maintaining proper equilibrium of these adrenal hormones.

Depending on the symptoms of stress a patient presents, I recommend the following, with the first two tests being the most important.

1. The *Koenigsberg* is a urine test for adrenal insufficiency. The procedure assesses urinary chloride levels and gives a measurement of sodium excretion. The goal is to assess subclinical stages of high or low adrenal function due to prolonged periods of stress.
2. A timed test that checks saliva for cortisol over the day (morning, afternoon, evening and night).
3. A DHEA test performed on saliva, with the sample taken at home overnight.
4. A catecholamine urine test to determine levels of adrenalin. Urine catecholamine testing measures the total amount of catecholamines released in twenty-four hours.

Since hormone levels may fluctuate significantly during this period, the urine test may detect excess production that is missed by a blood test.

I've little doubt that ten years from now these tests will be part of common clinical practice. For now, you can get a head start on them with at-home testing for antioxidant status, vitamin C levels and adrenal function in my test kit. Not only does testing determine your free radical levels, it also helps determine whether you're taking enough antioxidants—or too many. It can help you evaluate your current proximity to your personal health threshold. Testing will indicate the effectiveness of your diet or of your antioxidant supplements, effectiveness that might be quite different from the manufacturers' claims, thus allowing you to "debunk the junk" that is sometimes part of the natural health industry and avoid spending money unnecessarily on antioxidant foods or products that aren't working for you.

Lastly, consistently abnormal indicators—whether you observe your body's visible signs or monitor the results of at-home tests—should prompt you to further investigation. Fortunately, there are now a host of highly sensitive tests available through health-care providers. That's where we'll turn next.

LABORATORY TESTS

Like mainstream medical doctors, practitioners of the art of natural medicine believe it important to screen for diseases, though we choose to respond by using natural and non-invasive alternatives instead of prescription drugs or surgery. We aspire to do more than that though. We aspire to identify the less life-threatening glitches and minor upsets in our patients' biochemistry long before disease has a chance to set in, investigating underlying cause rather than current symptom expression.

FUNCTIONAL TESTS

Some practitioners such as myself refer to this process as *functional* testing. By *functional* we mean much the same as *holistic*—concerned with underlying causes rather than symptoms.

Testing for free radicals tells us about our current health status, but also discloses the *potential* for developing specific diseases. Relatively few mainstream doctors run tests on free radical levels, generally because they wouldn't have a solution for the problem once the results came back, and their patients would not—not at that moment, anyway—qualify for drugs or surgical intervention should the tests indicate high levels of free radicals. Nor do many mainstream doctors routinely tell their patients to take antioxidants, exercise more regularly, eat more vegetables and cut out as many stressful factors as possible. Medical practitioners are focused on ways to save your life when you're in trouble. Their tests are to that end—necessary in an emergency room but not able to keep you well throughout your life—or when dealing with a chronic disease. On the other hand, natural practitioners—and many holistically oriented MDs—are interested in keeping you alive, healthy and in tip-top shape *in the long term*.

Natural-medicine practitioners are now able to avail themselves of many well-researched and accurate laboratory tests, such as nutritional status testing, exact vitamin and mineral cellular status, metabolic analysis, neurochemistry analysis, salivary hormone testing, digestive function assessment,

Genetic predisposition isn't necessarily destiny: just because your mother has asthma or your father is suffering from Alzheimer's doesn't mean that you will succumb to either or both afflictions. Your genetics do dictate, however, that if you reach the boiling point on a constant basis, free radicals will cause you to develop whatever your genes may have in store for you in the realm of disease. Another reason to know your antioxidant health status.

genetic evaluation, antioxidant status and many more. None of these tests were manufactured or discovered by practitioners of natural medicine or by the manufacturers of natural medicines either. They were invented by research scientists curious about the biological processes of the body.

For those of you who want to know more about this enormously important but still breaking science, or who want to bring this subject to your doctor's attention, I've created Appendix D at the end of the book. There we'll look carefully at the validity of these tests, how to interpret them and which of them are accepted by mainstream medical practitioners. If the discussion in Appendix D intrigues you but exceeds your taste for technical and medical issues, I urge you to search actively for a practitioner versed in free radical testing and up on the latest free radical–antioxidant science.

MY TOP INVESTIGATIVE TESTS

In the table below, I list four functional tests for biomarkers that point to some *causes* of free radical accumulation. These are the tests I perform most often for patients in my practice. You can ask your doctor to run them as add-ons to the more standard disease-screening protocols. If your doctor dismisses these tests too quickly, he or she may simply not know about them or understand how to run them. If you need to find someone who *does* know how to run and interpret them for you, you can contact any large laboratory that processes these tests (see Appendix D) and ask them for access to their database of the doctors who offer them.

FUNCTIONAL TEST NO. 1: TOXINS

A combination test to determine the levels of heavy metals (including arsenic, mercury, aluminum, cadmium and lead) from a toxin panel on hair, blood and urine.

Reason for this test: Sometimes our bodies are bombarded with toxins, which are true obstacles to cure. They cause extreme free radical burden.

FUNCTIONAL TEST NO. 2: LIVER FUNCTION

Get a comprehensive test for liver function that checks levels of liver enzymes known as AST, ALT, ALP and GGT. When enzymes are elevated, conventional understanding is that the liver is toxic, infected or degenerative. The best possible analysis is achieved when the tests above are combined with detoxification challenge tests and genetic tests that look at your genetic potential for detoxification.

Reason for this test: All blood is purified through the liver. When the liver isn't functioning well, free radicals accumulate instead of being eliminated.

FUNCTIONAL TEST NO. 3: HEART HEALTH

Test a series of cardiovascular markers: triglycerides, total cholesterol, HDL, LDL, VLDL, apolipoproteins [apo A, apo B, Lp(a)], homocysteine, hs-CRP, HbA1c, fibrinogen, Lp-PLA2 (PLAC test for ischemic stroke), NT-ProBNP, skin sterols (correlating to cholesterol deposition).

Reason for this test: According to the American Heart Association, this year in the United States alone, 1.2 million people are expected to have a new or recurrent coronary attack. As many as 3 to 4 million Americans may have ischemic episodes without knowing it. In Canada, about 70,000 people a year have heart attacks. Most alarming: about 50 per cent of heart attacks are *silent or unexpected*.

Most doctors have access to all of these tests with the exception of the skin sterol test.

FUNCTIONAL TEST NO. 4: FULL NUTRITIONAL STATUS

Undergo a comprehensive nutritional test on blood, saliva and urine that evaluates overall nutritional status, provides insight into disease risk and assesses the functional needs of many vitamins and amino acids for body and brain.

Reason for this test: to help you determine what's missing from your diet and what you need to do, beyond taking antioxidants, to avoid disease.

Toxins

If politicians get themselves tested for heavy metals just to make a political point, then perhaps so should you. The concern is that lead, mercury and arsenic exposure through common household products and children's toys as well as the fish we eat and the water we drink can increase our heavy metal (and directly our free radical) load. If this is found to be so in your case, it is correctible with the appropriate chelation and antioxidant treatment.

Liver Function

When you are exposed to more toxicity than your liver can handle, or are born with less of an ability to clear toxins than average, or have a medical history of liver infection or other affliction, this test will help you and your health provider better understand what antioxidants can do for you to help clean up the free radical debris resulting from a liver that is not functioning optimally.

Heart Health

New tests may be developed from scratch in laboratories, but it's quite common for new uses for existing tests to evolve through clinical practice. This is how a test called the high-sensitivity C-reactive protein (hs-CRP) test, which appears as part of Functional Test No. 3, has become increasingly used for predicting the risk of heart disease. Its original purpose was to assess infection or inflammation associated with disease. I believe that everyone should have this test as part of their regular screening. It's a decent predictor of free radical damage and a good predictor of the injury to the cardiovascular and artery lining. If this inflammation is found to be high, cholesterol is prone to deposit at the site of injury in order to get the healing process started. Next comes clogging of the arteries.

You'll see that a group of biomarkers called apolipoproteins form part of my recommended Functional Test No. 3. Ask your doctor to run these tests when he or she is ordering up your cholesterol tests. Physicians rarely test the apolipoprotein biomarkers, but researchers who conducted a Mayo Clinic study have argued that these specific apolipoprotein components may be better markers for risk of heart disease than cholesterol itself, and researchers at Johns Hopkins have suggested that apo A-I and apo B are better indicators of premature coronary atherosclerosis than markers such as LDL cholesterol.

If you have a personal or family history of heart disease, there is no question that you must actively learn about *all* of the ways in which you can stay on top of good heart health. Tests in Functional Test No. 3, when carried out together, provide a comprehensive look at the health of your heart and blood vessels. This is especially important as a first step in the use of antioxidants for preventing the progression of disease. If the results should be abnormal, they'll be compelling evidence that you must maintain a good diet and exercise routine. You'll also want to supplement with a high-dose omega-3 fatty acid (5 g twice daily on average), take extra ACES and supplement with high doses of B complex, including folic acid and B_{12}. In some cases it may be very helpful to take an 81 mg Aspirin tablet daily.

Full Nutritional Status

The NutrEval test offered by Genova Diagnostics is the Cadillac of nutritional assessments, a tool that saves a clinician from having to guess about your current nutritional status and nutrient demands. It looks at how you metabolize of thirty-nine key organic acids in order to evaluate gastrointestinal function, cellular energy production, neurotransmitter processing and functional need for vitamins, minerals and other cofactors. It also evaluates amino acids, measuring thirty-eight of them to evaluate dietary protein adequacy, digestion, absorption, amino acid transport, metabolic impairments and nutritional deficits, including essential vitamins and minerals. It assesses omega-3 fatty acids and levels of inflammation in the body. It will also identify short-term toxic metal exposure and evaluate intracellular nutrient mineral status.

CANCER AND AIDS: A CAUTION

Cancer and AIDS are diseases notorious for their indiscriminate toll on human life. Both diseases respond to some degree to antioxidant therapy. I say "to some degree" because I must warn those who are affected not to begin arbitrarily supplementing their diet with everything under the sun that can provide an immune boost. It is not always the right thing to do to boost your immune system—to supplement with antioxidants when your free radical levels are too low. In cancer and AIDS, there are times when by virtue of treatment your free radical levels actually get too low. There are other times, such as during chemotherapy, when free radicals are deliberately high, and we don't want to counteract the potency of the chemotherapy by overdosing on antioxidants. For those of you afflicted with these diseases or who are caring for cancer or AIDS patients, please consult with your primary health-care practitioner.

Now that we've learned about the importance of balancing antioxidants and free radicals, and have learned how to test ourselves for them, what do we do with that knowledge?

PART TWO

—

THE ACTION PLAN

—

CHAPTER 6

THE FOUR Rs

I promised at the start of this book that I was going to offer you a simple action plan that would lead to better health. To this point, we've been reviewing the whys of sickness and health—the basic facts that we must understand if we're going to make the right choices. From here on, we're going to look at the hows.

When I was in high school, our vice-principal would stand smiling in the hallway as his students trooped in every morning and call out, "Remember, you Runnymede Redmen! Respect, responsibility and rights!" He embodied a fourth R without having to speak it: reciprocity. He always gave back. I still have a soft spot for his four Rs.

The next time I came across the concept of life lived according to four Rs, it was while attending a continuing education seminar sponsored by Metagenics, a leading vitamin and nutrition supplement company whose slogan is "unlocking the secrets of genetic potential through nutrition." Metagenics' four Rs were all about helping define ways in which people could avoid exceeding their human health threshold. If you've read this far, you know that our objective is to discover what it is in our diet, lifestyle, genetic code and environment that needs to be mitigated and monitored so as *not* to push us over our threshold into a state of disease. In the spirit of my old vice-principal and with gratitude to Metagenics, I've come up with *my* fours Rs to help guide you through the action plan. Turn to them whenever you need to treat a condition you've developed or any time you fall off the wagon and want to get back to a state of optimal health.

THE FIRST R: REMOVE OBSTACLES TO CURE

The first of the four Rs reminds us that our most important challenge is to *remove* obvious obstacles to cure—health roadblocks that impede the body's natural defences, and so push our health status to the threshold and beyond. Free radicals are of course the primary obstacle, but before we start taking more antioxidants, we're going to remove the sources of free radicals. For simplicity's sake, here are six ways we go about this first important step.

1. Remove Bad Habits

There are certain choices we make on a regular basis, more from habit than anything else. Some of these choices are bad for us and we know it. Smoking is a classic example, and I'm sure I need say nothing more about it here. Another is excessive alcohol consumption. Modern research encourages the moderate consumption of alcohol—red wine especially—but you should limit yourself to one glass of wine per day if you are a woman and not pregnant (don't drink at all if you are pregnant) and two glasses per day if you're a man. These limits are based on scientifically secure findings and demand your serious attention.

Let's also remember that one of the most destructive habits is the habit of doing nothing; so remove yourself from the couch and get going!

2. Remove Unnecessary Injury

You'll remember my example of Lance Armstrong, the remarkable American athlete whose cancer I suggested might have been linked to overexertion. But even if you're not pedalling through the Alps, you can still overdo your enthusiasm for fitness. That's why, when we come to Chapter Eleven, "Your Personal Antioxidant Exercise Plan," the emphasis will be on a balanced daily routine of weight-bearing and *non-impact* cardiovascular exercises. Injury is a major cause of joint inflammation, and inflammation of any kind means free radical damage.

3. Remove Radiation

When we looked at the sources of free radical accumulation, high on the list was ultraviolet radiation from the sun. Avoid it by covering up and using as chemical-free a sunblock as you can find. As to the grade, this depends on your skin type, but in general I recommend SPF 45. It's true that one of the best ways of getting the antioxidant vitamin D is through sun exposure: experts recommend spending twenty minutes a day uncovered in the sun at non-peak hours. Even if you are diligent with sunscreen, chances are you'll get enough contact with direct sunlight to maximize your natural vitamin D.

If you live in a house with a basement, I urge you to have your residence tested for radon gas. Testing is the only way to detect radon levels.

And then there's your cell phone. I know you can't live without it. But it's not worth dying for either. Strike a reasonable balance. In Canada, unlike many countries, we have a wonderful land-line system. Don't use your cell phone when a call from an ordinary phone will do—and often costs you less. While research into this grey area goes forward, why not let others be the guinea pigs?

For more on the dangers of these and other forms of radiation, see Appendix B.

4. Remove Stress

When we examined the causes of free radical burden, you may have been surprised to find mental and emotional stress is linked to changes in our bodies at the molecular level. But the effects of stress are real, and as we're going to see, there are healthy ways of reducing it. It's an important part of our action plan and I'm going to devote a whole chapter to it.

5. Remove Uncertainty

When you're in a strange town and using a map, you simply can't determine which way to go until you determine where you are. In the same way, you cannot make wise decisions about your health without learning something about your present health status. That's why I devoted a chapter to testing your antioxidant status and your free radical levels. Remove uncertainty and go forward with confidence.

6. Remove Toxins

Clearly we want to remove damaging contaminants from our surroundings and our bodies. There are two ways of accomplishing this: by avoiding these toxins and by getting rid of the ones that have taken up unwelcome residence in us. I'm going to devote the next chapter to detoxification and outline a safe and effective plan to achieve it.

THE SECOND R: REPLENISH

When you've removed the obstacles to cure and lowered the burden to your health by removing sources of free radicals, the next step is to replenish yourself. We recognize that once our threshold is exceeded, free radicals accumulate and many parts of the body suffer. In Chapter Ten, "Your Personal Antioxidant Supplement Plan," I'm going to describe this critical replenishment process—the general system boost you're going to give your body by restoring these nutrients and food factors in conjunction with antioxidant therapy. As an extreme example, think of a starving African child, bloated from malnutrition. This child wouldn't benefit from antioxidant and mineral supplementation until she has been fed properly on the building blocks of life, with a diet of protein, fat and carbohydrates.

THE THIRD R: REGENERATE

If replenishment is a general system overhaul—a restoration of crucial biological material—regeneration refers to cellular antioxidant support. Regeneration of your cells once you've dealt with the harmful free radical load requires a short-term therapeutic routine of supplementation with high-dose antioxidants in order to power a therapeutic response. We'll talk about that too in Chapter Ten.

THE FOURTH R: REPAIR

Our bodies are in a continuing process of damage and repair. Since our cells are constantly undergoing damage from free radicals, they also constantly need reparative maintenance. The repair stage is the antioxidant support that helps to maintain your body in an optimal state of health. It also has a place in Chapter Ten.

Remove. Replenish. Regenerate. Repair. Not as grand sounding as my old vice-principal's four Rs, but as important for your health as his four were for the spirit of us Runnymede Redmen. Now let's learn how to put them into practice.

CHAPTER 7

YOUR DETOXIFICATION PLAN

The first of the four Rs is *Remove*. Detoxifying is my topic in this chapter and the number one step in our plan. But a critical part of detoxification is not encountering toxins in the first place.

THE FIRST LINE OF DEFENCE

So here again is our parade of villains, this time with some advice on how to avoid them.

Plastics

Plastics release some dangerous stuff, and many plastics are now implicated in causing cancer. Plastics should not be heated nor kept near us, especially in the first days after purchase when they are "off-gassing." Especially notorious and worthwhile avoiding altogether are the PVC plastics #3, #6 and #7 (you'll usually find the number grade on the bottom of the container). Alternatives such as stainless steel and glass can readily replace them—and these alternatives are finally making their way back into the marketplace due to public awareness and concern. If you *must* use plastic, then the following are the "better" plastics:

- #1 Polyethylene terephthalate (PET or PETE), *the most common and easily recycled plastic for bottled water and soft drinks, has also been considered the most safe. But if there is a hint of plastic smell or taste in your water, don't drink it. Avoid exposing bottled water to heat, which enhances the leaching of plastic chemicals. Always ask your retailer how long bottled water has been sitting on the shelves and under what conditions and use the water you buy quickly: chemicals may leach from the plastic during storage. Slightly higher concentrations of PET have been found in still water as opposed to sparkling water samples, but no one yet understands why. The jury is still out on all plastics.*
- #2 High-density polyethylene.
- #3 Low-density polyethylene.
- #4 Polypropylene.

Automotive Toxins

Vehicles spew about seventy million tons of global-warming pollution daily into the thin shell of our atmosphere. If you live in a city, it's hard to avoid the toxicity of automobile emissions. The most practical advice I can offer is to be part of the solution and rely as much as you can on public transportation. We would all benefit from the widespread adoption of the new generation of low-emission vehicles.

Other Chemicals

"Other chemicals" refers to the wide range of substances including industrial gases, synthetic dyes, pigments, resins, synthetic rubbers, artificial and synthetic fibres, filaments, pesticides, fertilizers and other agricultural chemicals, paints, coatings, adhesives, soaps, cleaning compounds and personal care products. Common pollutants emitted from chemical manufacturing facilities include sulphur oxides, nitrogen oxides, volatile organic compounds (VOCs), particulate matter, carbon monoxide, carbon dioxide and dioxins.

We are constantly exposed to toxic chemicals every day through commonly used products in the home, such as perfumes, shampoos, air fresheners and even furniture and appliances. Many harmful chemicals are deliberately added to health and beauty products to improve our perception of them. What most of us don't know is that we're applying a little bit of cancer to our face along with the pretty purple hue of an eyeliner. That's why you should avoid topical use of the ingredient butylated hydroxyanisole (BHA), also found in eye shadow, concealer and lipstick; it's been shown to have carcinogenic and liver-toxic effects. Coal tar, found in shampoos, conditioners and bath oils, is known to cause immune system toxicity and organ system impingement.

Clearly, the best detoxification program is to *avoid* these things. As consumers, we must train ourselves to read *and* understand the labels on products meant for external application as well as those meant for ingestion.

Make sure that you keep your home as chemical free as possible. Use cleaners that are eco-friendly. If a chemical can burn a hole in your grass, what's it doing to your lungs and nervous system? Bleach and harsh chemicals facilitate the creation of more resistant and virulent strains of viruses and bacteria; using them for daily cleaning is unnecessary. Daily cleaning with water and vinegar easily suffices. Use those harsher chemicals and abrasives once every two weeks if you must. A common trick is to add baking soda or toothpaste to your water and vinegar when you need an abrasive for surfaces such as kitchen sinks and stove tops.

You should apply the same vigilance to your personal hygiene products and toiletries. For example, purchase aluminum-free deodorant; there are serious neurotoxicity concerns about aluminum salts.

Water and Air

Have your water tested for chlorine and chloroform, which are by-products of municipal water purification, and residual bacteria, as well as the heavy metals mercury, barium and arsenic. I guarantee that you are going to find that your water supply is contaminated at some level, and I recommend that everyone uses a reverse osmosis water purifier in their home. I use a water system that promises to remove every contaminant to 0.0005 microns in size, which happens to be smaller than a virus.

I also recommend an attachment on your shower to remove chlorine, because chlorine damages and dries out the skin and is absorbed into the body.

If you can afford it, install a high-efficiency particulate air (HEPA) filter into your general ventilation to remove the environmental toxins that inevitably make their way in from the outdoors. This includes smog and the seasonal allergens that so trouble some of us.

Heavy Metals

Mercury

Most of us have had exposure to mercury through mercury amalgam dental fillings—the "silver" filling most of us have in our mouths. And the exposure poses surprising danger to our health. If you're concerned about mercury fillings, what should you do?

First, you should know that good old gold and porcelain inlays, onlays and crowns, although more expensive than amalgam, are just as good or better and don't pose the toxic danger.

Second, you should consider having your amalgam fillings replaced. For the record, I'm having my own amalgam fillings removed, one at a time at two-month intervals. As part of this program, I take metal "chelators" (binders and removers of heavy metals) and antioxidants such as alpha-lipoic acid; antioxidants also help remove mercury from the body. Even a dentist using a rubber dam and great suction will still have you inhaling the deadly vapour that arises from drilling out this hardened quicksilver.

To rid the body of mercury, I recommend either oral, or, if necessary, intravenous chelation therapy, supplements such as alpha-lipoic acid, cilantro tincture, chlorella algae powder and garlic, as well as various amino acids, and I also recommend eating foods rich in vitamin E. I can't recommend specific dosages here because the proper dose is *so* dependant on age and body weight.

You can lower your mercury levels from other sources over time by avoiding shark, swordfish, king mackerel and tilefish, all of which have unacceptably high levels of mercury.

Arsenic

Arsenic can make its way into our drinking water. It makes sense to have your water tested by a private laboratory. If arsenic or other contaminants are at elevated levels, invest in a reverse osmosis water filter, as I recommended above, or a water distiller. I use a reverse osmosis unit that can be mounted under the sink. It works silently and is self-sterilizing. You need change the filter only about once a year, depending on how hard the filter must work to keep your water clean.

Also, stop smoking. There is a *huge* arsenic exposure from cigarette smoke. If testing detects significant arsenic levels in your body, I recommend a product called Bio-Chelat, which forms a sturdy bond with many heavy metals, including arsenic and mercury, and pulls them out of the body. And also Cell Rejuvenate, which contains fulvic acid and is good for cell support during heavy metal chelation.

Lead

To avoid lead contamination over time, I recommend you avoid certain crystal lead-lined decanters, renovating old houses (pre-1960s especially) painted with lead paint, dust (yes, the stuff on your bedroom floor often contains environmental lead) and corroded plumbing or lead-soldered plumbing, as well as certain pesticides and fertilizers.

Animal studies have shown that antioxidants—vitamins B_6, C and E; zinc; taurine; *N*-acetylcysteine and alpha-lipoic acid—either alone or in conjunction with standard chelating agents, are very helpful in removing lead from the systems of animals exposed to this toxic metal.

The Bad in the Good: Fish Oil

We're not only bombarded by toxins, we're also bombarded with advice on how to live longer and healthier lives—and here I am doing my best to contribute to the latter.

One of the new certainties of health care is that everyone should be consuming omega-3 fatty acids as part of their daily routine. But just as good things such as sunblocks can smuggle bad things into our lives, omega-3 supplementation carries risks.

Omega-3 fatty acids occur naturally in some nuts and seeds and fish, especially fatty fish such as mackerel, and are now known to provide protection against cardiovascular disease and much else. As a result—and because not everyone wants to or can eat a lot of these foods—the consumption of fish oil in supplement form is on the rise.

But the world has become a toxic place. Fish live in water and waterways that have become sinks for these toxins. Once-pristine waters now contain contaminants such as mercury, dioxins and pesticides that ultimately become part of the food chain. The majority of these toxins accumulate over a lifetime in the fat of the host animal, with very little being excreted. Mercury escaping from an industrial facility or washed from the soil into the ocean can contaminate the algae on the ocean floor. These algae are food for small fish that are eaten, in turn, by larger fish that are eaten by even larger fish. When we eat tuna, a fish high on the food chain, the mercury that has worked its way up the food chain and concentrated in that fish is present at high levels. This concentrating effect is known as *bioaccumulation.*

With all our health awareness, we seem caught between protecting ourselves from heart disease and protecting ourselves from slow poisoning. But with a little care, we can accomplish this double feat by turning to purified, pharmaceutical-grade fish oil for our omega-3 supplementation.

North American labels don't offer enough information to consumers when it comes to fish oil supplements—that is, information about the type of fish, in which body of water it was caught, how the oils were processed and, most importantly, if the product has been tested by a third party to validate its quality and purity. But high-quality fish oil manufacturers voluntarily adhere to guidelines established by other regulatory bodies such as the World Health Organization (WHO) and the Council for Responsible Nutrition (CRN). The CRN fish oil monograph has set out the permissible limits of contaminants in fish oils.

In summary, you need to look at the total oxidation, or TOTOX, value of the fish oil in question: you want it to be low, as the more oxidation there is, the more free radical damage there is to the oil. The higher the TOTOX, the higher the chance the fish oil will do you more harm than good. The maximum you should tolerate is a level of 26. Acid value is another important measure, and you should look for oils that measure less than 3 mg potassium hydroxide (KOH) per gram. Rancidity factors such as the peroxide and anisidine values are also related to the oxidation of the oil and, if they are high, make it taste really bad: peroxide should be no higher than 5 milliequivalents (mEq) per kg and anisidine 20 mEq per kg. Heavy metals such as lead, cadmium, mercury and arsenic should be less than 0.1 m per kg in your chosen fish oil. If there are dioxins and furans, they need to be at levels less than 2 per gram. Lastly, PCBs should be less than 0.09 mg per kg. These polychlorinated biphenyls aren't produced any longer in North America, but they are still found in the environment and can cause hormonal disturbances.

The term "pharmaceutical grade" when applied to fish oil refers to quality and purity standards that comply with the CRN monograph. Since compliance with the CRN monograph is not mandatory by law, consumers can be fooled by misleading label claims. The only true assurance for quality and purity comes from companies that have each and every batch of finished product tested and validated by a third-party laboratory. Here are the most common misleading label statements:

Pharmaceutical Grade
Many products make this statement but have no proof as in third-party testing. No laws exist to govern this statement. Question your supplier on the product manufacturer's basis for making this claim.

Third-Party Tested

Some products have been tested but not by independent labs. Some companies will submit several batches for third-party testing, yet only make available to consumers the test results that meet the grade. If a product indicates that it has been tested by a third-party, consumers should ask the manufacturer for the report on a specific batch number.

Toxin Free

This is perhaps one of the most misleading statements found on fish oil labels. Toxins exist in all foodstuffs, especially fish. The highest-quality fish oils have undergone purification to "reduce" contaminants down to CRN-compliant levels. No product on the market contains zero contaminants. Manufacturers that make this statement are purposely trying to be misleading or simply do not understand fish oil processing.

Highly purified fish oils from some manufacturers have been shown to be free of any detectable level of such contaminants as mercury. Here are a few questions to ask that may help you improve your chances of purchasing fish oil with reduced toxicity.

- *Is the product in a dark bottle to eliminate light oxidation? If not, free radicals may already be accumulating in the oil.*
- *Has the product been submitted for third-party testing. If so are these reports available to consumers? Badger your natural health-care provider and health-food store proprietor for this information.*
- *From which fish is the oil taken? (Herring, for example, is known to be relatively free of contaminants.)*
- *Where was the fish caught?*

> • *How have the fish oils been refined?*
> • *Did the manufacturer follow the CRN and WHO guidelines?*

My brand preference is NutraSea omega-3 fish oil because it meets all of the above criteria. I have supplemented my son's diet with it since he was six months old. Before that, he got it through his mother's breast milk, and before that through my wife's diet. My daughter, now six months old, is next.

I recommend that everyone take this supplement. The average dose is 1 teaspoon twice daily.

Food Additives

A simple rule about additives is to avoid those found in the charts in Appendix C. Not only are they among the most questionable additives, but they are also used primarily in foods of low nutritional value.

If the food or product in question says on its label that it contains artificial colour, colour, food colouring, natural colour (unless specified from the natural source such as beet juice) and any other term you deem an imaginative synonym—avoid it. These foods are usually bad for you for other reasons anyhow. The generally accepted avoid list includes Blue No. 1, Blue No. 2, Green No. 3, Red No. 3, Red No. 40, Yellow No. 5, Yellow No. 6, Orange B and Citrus Red No. 2.

However, some food additives are not suspect, such as annatto extract, beta-carotene, beet powder, canthaxanthin, carrot oil, fruit juice, grape colour extract, grape skin extract, paprika, paprika oleoresin, riboflavin, saffron, turmeric and vegetable juices.

Sugar and Salt

We talked about this merry pair in Chapter Three, but there's no harm in giving them one more bad review. According to a new report issued by the non-profit Center for Science in the Public Interest, eating too much salt is boosting our blood pressure and prematurely killing roughly 150,000 of us each year in North America. We are now consuming on average about 4,000 mg (4 g) of sodium per day—about twice the recommended amount. That's easy to believe when you consider that 5 g of salt is only a level teaspoon.

When it comes to sugar, we need a bit of it daily to feed our brains, but we are not hummingbirds. Refined sugar in our diet is one of the leading causes of inflammation, obesity, diabetes, heart disease and, of course, free radical accumulation. Sugar is extremely high in empty calories, suppresses the immune system, distorts our brain chemistry, causes blood discrepancies and leads to premature aging and a more rapid decline in health. Consume no more than 25 g a day—the equivalent of 5 level teaspoons—above and beyond what you naturally get from whole foods. More than a day's allowance—about 7 teaspoons—is found in one can of pop.

In general, we can avoid food additive risks by avoiding food additives. If you strive to eat and drink only organic, chemical-free foods high in oxygen radical absorbance capacity (ORAC), you'll spare your body enormous effort and stress. I'll have more to say about that in Chapter Nine, when we set up your nutritional routine.

Prescription Drugs

My rule of thumb is quite simple. If you don't absolutely have to be on a medication long term, don't be. Try anything and everything else that is proven effective to manage your health issue. Have you appropriately and safely tried all other alternatives to the pharmaceutical? In some cases—cancer and emergency surgery and certain other grave situations—prescription medication is a godsend. But in many other chronic conditions, we rely on drugs because we are uneducated as to the alternatives, or too lazy to stick to them. If it's absolutely necessary that you take or remain on some of the more common prescription medication, I suggest that you seriously consider supplementing with the antioxidant that best helps to curtail the side effects of that prescription medication. Discuss this with your natural health-care provider.

DETOXIFY

We've looked at how we can avoid ingesting toxins and touched on how to get rid of toxins in special cases. But what about the body's inevitable accumulation of toxic burden from daily living? How can we deal with that?

The Body's Natural Detoxifier: The Liver

We're exposed to a myriad of foreign chemicals, but other toxins—called endotoxins—are actually produced within the body. Our bodies signal an overload of toxic substances in many ways: headache; muscle and joint pain; fatigue; irritability; depression; mental confusion; gastrointestinal tract irregularities; cardiovascular irregularities; flu-like symptoms; or allergic reactions, including hives, stuffy or runny nose, sneezing and coughing.

The liver, the central toxic-waste site of the body, works hard every second of the day and night to sieve these toxins. It is also a metabolic factory where everything—the air we breathe, the food we eat, the medicines we take—is transformed. It's responsible for breaking down and packaging up proteins, carbohydrates and fats and, as if that isn't enough, it synthesizes bile and glycogen (the principle form in which sugar is stored) and the blood proteins that the body uses for energy and metabolism.

In the process, the liver is guilty—and who can blame it?—of accumulating free radicals. We can hardly expect a busy factory not to produce some smoke.

The liver is capable of healing and regenerating itself, but an overloaded liver leaks poisons into the bloodstream that can injure organs and diminish our health. We need to help it along with a routine, health-optimizing "spring cleaning"—the important next step in our program.

Cleansing

The health food industry didn't make up this notion. Cleansing, along with detoxification, is pure biological science. While you're reading these lines, your body is conducting thousands, if not millions, of intricate biochemical processes for the sole purpose of keeping you alive. A natural cleanse is meant to help your body with this process of toxin clearance. Cleansing programs are designed to aid the body's natural detoxification process— when that process is not overly burdened.

You've probably heard about some cleansing routines—the water and juice fasts, which supposedly work on the principle that the body will heal itself when the "stress" of digestion is eliminated. Such cleanses may do more harm than good. The natural liver processes I've just described are not only energy intensive, but are also dependent on adequate levels of supporting nutrients. A water fast that is totally devoid of energy sources or supportive nutrients may in fact *suppress* detoxification rather than enhance it. A juice fast may be effective since at least it provides some carbohydrates and other nutrients, but it's still deficient in vitamins, minerals and amino acids.

For these reasons, I advise you to *avoid* "drastic measures" like fasting.

Some popular cleansing protocols also recommend laxatives,

enemas or colonic irrigation to speed up the process. Dozens of books and hundreds of websites promote such "cleansing" regimens. Spas everywhere invite "cleansers" to spend thousands of dollars in exotic locations to expel their toxins in luxurious relaxation. These routines are often of little use and sometimes dangerous. And, like other fads, cleansing regimens promise quick weight loss that is always unsustainable. They're based on junk science rather than a true scientific understanding of how the body works. Worst of all, these extreme diets can cause serious side effects in vulnerable groups. Never do a cleanse of any kind, for instance, while pregnant. **Never put a child on a cleanse without expert advice.** Safe detoxification requires the use of therapeutic levels of well-researched antioxidants to facilitate and speed up the natural process.

I'm going to give you my prescription for a truly sensible and effective cleanse. Anyone between the ages of sixteen and one hundred can do it.

THE CLEANSE

This simple cleanse aids the liver's own complex detoxification pathways. Aim to do it twice annually; each time it will take you two to four weeks. For the duration of the cleanse, abstain from your personal antioxidant supplement routine, the one we're going to discuss in Chapter Ten. Your caloric intake along with the antioxidant-dense and nutrient-rich diet you'll be eating will drastically lower your need for supplementation. And remember I said we should do this to give your liver a break? Well that includes a break from your supplements, too.

Always check with a qualified health-care professional before doing this cleanse.

Special caution: especially do not proceed if you are pregnant or have diabetes.

The 7-Day Primer

While you are doing this primer, you should eat or drink nothing but what is recommended each day. The juices should be unrefined and as fresh as possible. Organically grown is most desirable. Drink about 175 ml (6 oz) at a time and not less than 7 or more than 10 servings in one day. The limit on the quantity of solids is described below. There is no limit on your consumption of pure water.

Juices for the 7-Day Primer

Day 1: Mix some turmeric into distilled water at a ratio of 1 mL (¼ tsp.) of the spice to 175 mL (6 ounces) of water. This cleanses the entire system while significantly reducing lingering inflammation.

Day 2: *Pineapple juice.* The bromelain enzyme in pineapple will cleanse the small intestine.

Day 3: *Lemon and water.* Acidifies, detoxifies and cleanses the liver.

Day 4: *Carrot juice.* Coats and lubricates the liver, lungs, kidneys and brain.

Day 5: *Beet juice.* Pulls toxins out of the liver into the bloodstream.

Day 6: *Green juices.* Cause an exchange of toxins across cell membranes, resulting in systematic flushing of the toxins out of the body. You can use a product called Greens Plus from Genuine Health or juice your own combination of equal parts of spinach, collards, arugula, parsley, kale and broccoli.

Day 7: *Decaffeinated green tea.* Detoxifies the body and primes your antioxidant status.

Daily Solids for the 7-Day Primer

1. 2 servings of ORAC fruits a day, eaten at least one hour before or after your grains and beans.
2. 1 L (4 cups) lightly steamed vegetables spread out throughout the day.
3. 125 mL (½ cup) of your choice of whole grain with half a cup of any bean or legume twice daily.
4. 250 mL (1 cup) One cup of organic yogurt, unflavoured and unsweetened, once daily.

So a day in your life while on the 7-day primer looks something like this:

Morning (on waking): 175 mL (6 oz.) of the day's indicated therapeutic liquid

Breakfast: ½ cup (125 mL) of whole grain and bean mixture with a topping of ½ cup (125 mL) yogurt and one serving of ORAC fruit

Mid-Morning: 175 mL (6 oz.) of the indicated liquid

Half an hour before lunch: 175 mL (6 oz.) of the indicated liquid

Lunch: 500 mL (2 cups) of lightly steamed vegetables

An hour after lunch: 175 mL (6 oz.) of the indicated liquid

Mid-Afternoon: 175 mL (6 oz.) of the indicated liquid

Dinner: 500 mL (2 cups) of lightly steamed vegetables. 125 mL (½ cup) of whole grain and bean mixture.

An hour after dinner: 175 mL (6 oz.) of the indicated liquid

Snack: 1 serving of ORAC fruit

Before bed: 175 mL (6 oz.) of the indicated liquid

The purpose of drinking the juices is to cleanse and detoxify the body. As a result, you might experience such common detoxification symptoms as mild nausea, loose bowels, headaches, muscular aches and pains, and skin rashes. You should not become alarmed by these symptoms. However, don't confuse these symptoms with true illness or infection. Consult with your doctor to be sure if any symptoms persist longer than the week you are on this primer.

On Day 8, move on to the *7- to 21-day brown rice cleansing diet* in conjunction with UltraClear Plus powder (a medical food developed by Metagenics and through natural heath-care practitioners and available in health food and nutrition stores).

The 7- to 21-Day Brown Rice Cleansing Diet

Sometimes our digestive organs need a break from the onslaught of aggravating foods and junk we put into them. Cleansing these organs allows them to function better and absorb nutrients more efficiently, thus making our bodies stronger and healthier. Do *not* attempt this diet without the supervision of your holistic health-care provider.

This diet will give you all the nutrition that you will need while your body cleanses and heals itself. You don't have to go hungry, and you don't have to count calories, or weigh food. You eat whenever you are hungry, and as often as you like. While on this diet, you may experience some weight loss.

Eat until you feel full, but not overly full. It is better to eat several small meals a day rather than three large ones.

Do not drink more than 115 mL (4 oz.) of liquids with your meals, as this dilutes the enzymes in the stomach needed to properly digest what you eat.

Try to keep the consumption of fruits separate from vegetables and rice, since some foods may be digested with greater ease and efficiency than others. This goes for fruit and vegetable juices as well.

What's Allowed on the Diet?

Quite a bit more than what's on the Primer, that's for sure.

- Brown rice, preferably organic.
- Fresh vegetables, any kind you like, lightly steamed. Onions are especially good for cleansing and are very sweet and tasty when steamed. Try a plate full with some brown rice and garlic.
- Fresh fruits, any kind, except oranges and orange juice, bananas and dried fruits. With fruits and vegetables, it is best to consume only organic produce whenever possible. However, as this is not always possible, *locally grown fruits and vegetables in season*, and wash them thoroughly before eating.
- Fresh garlic and ginger.
- Cayenne pepper and a non-salt herbal seasoning (such as Vegit).
- Vegetable and fruit juice. The best is fresh pressed from a juicer, otherwise, juices with no additives, sugar or chemicals, and little or no salt (a good variety are found in health food stores).
- Other foods that are allowed are lentils, rice cakes, sesame seeds, ocean-going fish, free-range organic chicken, hummus, tofu and tempeh.
- Absolutely no shellfish (shrimp, oysters, scallops, clams, lobster, etc.) or catfish.

EAT ONLY THESE FOODS (As much as you like!)

ORGANIC BROWN RICE

Rinse the rice first. Bring to a boil 500 mL to 560 mL (2 to 2¼ cups) of water per 250 mL (1 cup) of rice. Add the rice, turn the heat down to low, cover and simmer for 45 to 60 minutes. Do not stir while cooking. Herbs, spices and cooked onions can be added during the last 15 to 20 minutes of cooking time.

VEGETABLES (preferably organic)

All kinds of *fresh* vegetables can be eaten on this diet (except for corn and mushrooms, which often cause sensitivity and are highly allergenic). Make sure to wash them very well. They can be eaten raw, steamed or baked. Combine them with rice if you wish.

FRUITS (preferably organic)

All kinds of *whole* fruits can be eaten (except for bananas, oranges and some dried fruit). Make sure to wash them very well. Eat fruit raw. Eat fruit by itself, either one hour before or two hours after a meal.

MEAT AND BEANS (preferably organic)

Eat modest portions of meat and beans—enough to maintain your muscle mass but not so much as to burden your liver during the cleanse. For every kilogram of you weight, eat no more than 0.5 grams of ocean-going fish, organic free-range chicken, tofu, tempeh, hummus, lentils, red beans, mung beans and broad beans.

CONDIMENTS

Olive oil, lemon, pure herbs and spices that contain no salt or MSG, and flaxseed oil (which must be refrigerated, never heated and used within three weeks of opening it).

BEVERAGES

Filtered, distilled or spring water. Herbal teas, such as chamomile, mint, lemon. Vegetable and fruit juices—preferably freshly made. If you can't make them fresh, make sure they contain nothing other than 100 per cent juice—read your labels. Dilute juices half and half with water. Drink liquids half an hour before eating or one hour after.

MEDICAL FOOD

Have between ½ to 2 scoops of UltraClear or UltraClear Plus twice daily, dissolved in water and between meals, to aid in the clearance of toxins and to support your liver. It has all the antioxidants and vitamins you need in this cleansing diet to move out the "gunk."

This diet can be a very difficult venture. The more you stick with it, the better you will feel. Try your best and concentrate on what you are able to do, not what you aren't able to do.

After the seven to twenty-one days, it is important to come off the diet gradually. Don't overeat or splurge on junk food.

Start every day after you've finished your cleanse with a morning glass of room-temperature water into which you've squeezed half a lemon.

I also recommend taking the herb milk thistle for a month after you are done. Milk thistle possesses antioxidant properties and prevents damage to the liver, but, contrary to popular belief, is not so much a detoxifier as it is a rejuvenator. Most herbalists recommend the equivalent of 3 to 18 g of dried milk thistle fruit (wrongly known as seeds) per day for liver rehabilitative purposes. This is equal to 75 to 450 mg of the active ingredient, silymarin. After your cleanse, I suggest taking 100 mg of a standardized formula of milk thistle three times per day for the month to help the liver rejuvenate its cells.

SEEKING PROFESSIONAL ADVICE

With my own patients, the screening process that helps me decide whether to suggest a month-long detoxification usually entails a comprehensive evaluation, including a family and personal medical history, and a diet and nutrient record, either in journal or questionnaire form. Then I follow the evaluation by testing for how well the patient's liver enzymes are functioning. I then determine the specific toxin load using specialized testing for, say, heavy metals. I also perform other functional tests that assess an individual's ability to detoxify.

You don't have to run all these tests in order to begin a cleanse. On the other hand, it may be a good idea to have yourself assessed, because, even among healthy people, the efficiency of liver enzyme functions related to detoxification may vary by a factor of four to seven. Studies have shown that individuals who develop Parkinson's and Alzheimer's diseases often have a number of genetically impaired detoxification pathways. And children who are negatively affected by vaccinations may have inherent liver detoxification problems. In both cases, the pre-existing conditions may increase their susceptibility to the neurotoxic effects of free radicals.

The liver detoxifies in two chemical phases, the first a collection phase. If your liver is functioning well it takes those collected toxins and in phase two transforms them into water-soluble compounds that can be excreted through stool, urine or bile. We pee them out, poop them out, sweat them out and breathe them out. (If the liver isn't functioning well and removing toxins effectively, the body will store them in your nervous system and fat tissue, causing disease.) Antioxidants need to be replenished on a regular basis through dietary and supplement sources to improve liver function.

New studies of the liver's detoxification system suggest that if you're battling cancer, you may decide with a professional's help that a detoxification program is a prudent auxiliary strategy for your recovery.

In my clinic, successful detoxification or a simple cleanse always starts with UltraClear, one of the few natural detoxification medical foods on the market that has been tested and found to improve the liver's ability to clear caffeine, acetaminophen (Tylenol) and acetylsalicylic acid (Aspirin).

If you are suffering from a serious or chronic disease, my prescription for detoxification is this: Consult a professional who knows what they are doing. Then ensure that you are properly evaluated during the course of the protocol—often one month or longer. Typically, you'll feel worse before you feel better, since the toxins are recycled through your system before getting the boot.

NEXT STEPS

Of course all this removing should be followed by the other three Rs: replenishing, regenerating and repairing. That's what we're going to address with our supplementation program in Chapter Ten. Before we do, though, our action plan must address that other free radical accumulator—stress.

—

CHAPTER 8

YOUR STRESS REDUCTION PROGRAM

The time I've spent with thousands of patients in clinical practice has taught me about the enormous influence our minds exert on our health. The therapies I witnessed as a student of homeopathy often failed because of "obstacles to cure"—one of which was the patient's own mind. If the mind is resistant to healing or is subject to an underlying chemical condition preventing healing, the body will never attain health, but will decline due to disease and rapid aging.

When we looked at the underlying causes of free radical burden in Chapter Three, we discussed the intimate link between mind and body, the chemical pathways that are the brain's programmed response to stress and then how such responses generate free radicals. It follows that we may be able to use our minds to reprogram those ancient biochemical pathways so that everyday stressors don't crank up our systems to do battle with giant predators. In this chapter, I'm going to outline a simple program to relieve stress and the destructive reactions that stress triggers.

FUNCTIONAL MEDITATION

For myself and my patients, I've incorporated a number of "helpful thinking" techniques into what I call *functional meditation*. My program consists of several steps that work for me, and have worked for others.

Meditation is often thought to be the practice of attaining mental clarity by some kind of absolute mental decompression—perhaps the practice of thinking of nothing, long a technique of Theravada Buddhist monks and closely paralleled in other practices. Such meditation seems exceptionally difficult for the average North American. No doubt through years of practice, focus and dedicated concentration you can learn to shut off everything around you and in you at will. But for most of us, our brain seems determined to keep on going, asleep or awake.

It's a bit of a misconception, though, to define meditation solely as "thinking of nothing." Yes, meditation implies a clearing of the mind, but this can mean giving our minds a break from the daily mile-a-minute routine. The key to what I call functional meditation is *what* we think about and *how* we think about it— *the daily debrief.*

Functional meditation also aims to provide the tools by which to create our future, in fact, to *remember* our future; that is, to create defined and positive expectations—a desired state of mind—and to enjoy the result of healthy mind-body awareness.

We tend to get what we expect. If we simply hope, we invite opportunity for failure and leave fate to chance and circumstance. If on the other hand we make the effort to draw positive lessons from whatever happens, we always succeed.

This may seem facile, but it's not. We are the only conscious beings on earth with the ability to live under the influence of memory (not to be confused with instinct or learned behaviour). The pictures in our minds—our first kiss, our first car or our first born—are almost ineradicable. When we apply the functional meditation approach, we learn that, as far as our brain is concerned, there's no difference between what we've already experienced and what we *will* experience. The only thing that stands in the way of our getting exactly what we want is how much dedication we choose to put into the functional meditation exercise.

Of course, life can hit us at any time with the unexpected: none of us "wants" the car accident, hurricane, flood, brush with violence or death of a loved one that can hit us at any time. We can't plan for such events, but if you are diligent with your functional meditation routine, you'll have dealt with all the other stuff of life, and I think you'll find your reserves of emotional and spiritual energy are there to be drawn upon.

Here are the five steps of functional meditation.

STEP 1: The Life Agenda

Find some paper to write down the answers to your choice of three of the following six questions. Start smack in the middle of the page. Whatever comes first to mind is perfect.

- *What do I believe to be my purpose here on earth?*
- *What do I want to accomplish before my time is up?*
- *What do I want others to say about me in a eulogy?*
- *What is the point of my existence?*
- *In what way, so far, have I influenced the people close to me?*
- *Whenever I have an "ah-ha" moment—introspection that leads to clarity of purpose or some sort of "spiritual" revelation—the theme of it usually seems to be _____.*

There's no right or wrong answer to any of the above. Let whatever answers you have for three of these questions form the beginnings of what we'll call your *life agenda*. The many Okinawans who live to be one hundred and older, remaining healthy into advanced old age, have an equivalent to the idea of life agenda. They call it *ikigai*, translated as life purpose or that which makes one's life worth living.

Over the days, weeks, months and even years to come, you could do worse than to evolve your *ikigai* on this single piece of paper. Let the words and sentences that define your life agenda radiate out web-like from the point at which you started today. Consider this work personal, so don't leave it out in the open. Consider it, in fact, nothing less than sacred. Don't underestimate the power of this step and skip over it just because it may seem challenging. This is a crucial part of a work-in-progress and, if you do derive from it all the potential it holds, it will remain a work-in-progress until the day you die.

Another way to describe a life agenda is to consider it a legacy. How do you want others to remember you? What imprint do you intend to leave on this planet? Once you've considered the answers to these two questions (they may not come to you overnight), you'll find it easier to formulate your goals in greater detail.

Here are a few questions that may help you gain perspective in areas that many people consider important.

ARTISTIC:

Do you want to achieve any artistic goals? If so, what?

ATTITUDE:

Is any part of your mindset holding you back? Is there any part of the way that you behave that upsets you? If so, set a goal to improve your behaviour or find a solution to the problem.

CAREER:

What occupation do you want to pursue? What level do you want to reach in your career?

EDUCATION:

Is there any knowledge you want to acquire? What information and skills will you need to achieve other goals?

FAMILY:

Do you want to be a parent? If so, how are you going to be a good parent? How do you want to be seen by a partner or by members of your extended family?

FINANCIAL:

How much do you want to earn and by what point?

PHYSICAL:

Are there any athletic goals you want to achieve? Do you want good health well into old age? What steps are you going to take to achieve these goals?

PLEASURE:

How do you want to enjoy yourself?

PUBLIC SERVICE:

Do you want to make the world a better place? If so, how?

STEP 2: Long-, Medium- and Short-Term Goals

The importance of a one-page description of our life agenda is that we can extrapolate from this agenda to formulate *long-term goals*. Becoming more aware over time of your life agenda is going to make fulfilling your dreams *so* much easier and take away a tremendous amount of uncertainty and stress. Studies show that when we write things down after mulling them over, we are 90 per cent more likely to follow through with action designed to achieve those goals.

You must now put out feelers to test the logic of these long-term goals. Do they support your life agenda? Ideally, setting such goals is a sequential, focused process, though we humans tend to be dynamic beings who lead dynamic lives that are seldom either focused or sequential. We're prone, for example, to establish goals based on the short term, and then get caught up in a decision-making sequence that doesn't fit into the big picture. "I really want that car," we say. "Gosh, I better work hard to get it. That means I'll have to stay at the office late every night to rack up overtime hours. Hey, wait a minute! My priority right now is to meet a life partner. If I always stay late, I'll never meet new people and I'll never get married. Do I want a nice car or a soulmate? What a crazy question! Okay, for now I may just have to accept that I'm the driver of a beat-up old Ford Escort and go out during the week and enjoy a social life."

All this is to say that we need to establish a big picture—that's where the life agenda comes in—before we can extrapolate our long-term goals. If driving an expensive car doesn't seem to have anything to do with our long-term goals (which should flow out of our life agenda), then we can redirect our energies and funds elsewhere. If such a car *does* seem a necessary part of our plan, we go for it. Unless we make this effort to determine what it is that we really want from our future, we can easily get caught up in the blind, chaotic push forward that adds to our uncertainty and stress.

Our long-term goals represent our personal quest, what we want to achieve in our lives as opposed to what gets done to us.

Our *medium-term goals* are derived from our long-term goals. In order to reach the long-term goals, we usually must reach the medium-term goals within a certain time frame. Our medium-term goals might encompass employment success, seeing our children successfully raised, building financial security, developing a particular skill, going back to school, perhaps even getting that new car.

Short-term goals are always the easiest to see, but seeing our priorities becomes easier once we've determined the long-term and medium-term goals. Short-term goals are like stepping stones that help us measure our progress. If one of your medium-term goals is to go back to school, your short-term goals might be to do the research and create a list of appropriate institutions, attend make-up classes regularly, participate in professional development and internship opportunities at a chosen institution, maintain a certain grade point average and stay up to date in your readings and assignments. It's easy to see how, without the longer-term planning, these short-term practical undertakings can have us zigzagging through life in a stressful manner and never getting as close as we otherwise could to accomplishing our life agenda. Some people are "lucky," but luck doesn't cut it for most of us.

STEP 3: The Congruency Check

It's critically important that we periodically check that we've remained on track to completing our life agenda—that our lives, in other words, are congruent with our goals. If we fail to do this, we can fall victim to complacency, which can grab us by the throat and stifle our life objectives.

The congruency check allows us to confirm our path and ensure that we're moving in the right direction. If in our daily practice we see that we're engaging regularly in behaviour that is *not* congruent with our life agenda, we immediately have to stop this behaviour or reframe our intended outcome. If for instance we want to get good marks in university but find that every night we're out at the bar, we need a reality check.

STEP 4: Editing

Most of us are all too aware of our shortcomings. Driven by our past experience, we sometimes convince ourselves that we are doomed to fail.

So imagine that you're a film editor and your life is the movie. You know the plot (your life agenda) and you've planned out your long-, medium- and short-term assemblages of scenes—your goals. Now imagine yourself moving through your entire day. Good editors have to acknowledge that unexpected things will occur. It turns out the director forgot to shoot a scene. And at one point a bunch of extras are looking in the camera, and you can't use that stuff. The whole movie's ruined, right?

Of course not. Your job as an editor is to rearrange the bits of film to create a movie that's as close as possible to the original vision. Your life agenda is unwavering; it's your interim goals that are flexible. Whatever reframing of your current expectations it takes to fulfill your life agenda is fine, as long as when you change paths you continue to head in the right direction. Preconceived notions of failure, defeat and fear need constant attention and editing so that life's curveballs—dropped scenes, bad performances, poor lighting conditions—are managed.

Here's how you can apply this editing process to your life.

STEP 5: The Five-Minute Daily Practice
The Opener

Begin by describing the life ahead of you as you want it to be, as laid out in your life agenda. Describe to yourself your dream home, family dynamics, ideal career or position, friendships, bank account and, most importantly, health. Describe these things to yourself as you *want* them to be, not as they are now. This description is a sort of mantra—an affirmation and realization of those things that you desire. Make this a routine opening to your daily practice. Repeat this mantra until it's so much a part of you that you don't need to be aware of what you are saying, and then move on in the daily routine.

The Day Ahead

Imagine the next twenty-four hours. Ask yourself: What is on my schedule today? What plans do I have? Who will I see? (Distinguish between people who offer you resistance and people whom you expect to be helpful.) Attempt to uncover your preconceived notions about your day. (Are you expecting to be bored, irritated, driven out of your mind by people's demands, or to be intrigued, stimulated and presented with challenges that you can meet?) Lay all this imagined material out as though it were a movie in your mind. Now watch it as if it were actually happening. See it, hear it, feel it and smell it. Every important part of your day and every routine should be considered. You only need to "watch" this *one* time.

Editing

Now ask yourself: What parts of the next twenty-four-hour hours do I *not* wish to be a part of my experience? What parts of this movie are incongruent with my life agenda and my long-, medium- and short-term goals? Like the film editor, watch the movie once more, this time *editing out the pieces that you would rather not experience.* Create replacement clips congruent with your goals for each of the segments you edited out and instruct your imaginary creative team to splice these into the movie instead.

As an example, you first picture yourself walking past your boss, sweating over what excuse to give him for not completing the task he assigned to you last week. Edit this out. Instead, imagine walking past your boss and greeting her in a warm and civil fashion and then proceeding to say, "By the way, I've been working hard to get that assignment to you in a timely manner. It should be done by Friday." With this scripting, not only are you off the hook, you have also set a goal. Now you can look forward to bumping into your boss rather than wondering how you're going to duck her. Find *all* of the parts to your day that you're worried about, fearful about, negative about, then edit them out and recreate them as your preferred ideal outcomes.

When you're finished (at first this may take a while to perfect and feel comfortable doing), play the newly edited movie over until it sticks with you. You'll prove to yourself that you will get what you expect. The more you do this, the more you'll see the power of projection and visualization.

Point Shifting

This is the ability to recognize unfavourable behaviour and immediately superimpose congruent behaviour. Here is how it works.

Our bodies behave in predictable ways when we are not in a resourceful place in our mind. Some of us bite our lip, some squirm in our seats, some bite our nails or pick at our skin. Others may twitch or jiggle one leg. Your body initiates these behaviours well before you're conscious of them. Your unconscious mind is aware of your surroundings and controls what you do before your conscious mind is invited to participate. Once your unconscious mind has picked up on an uncomfortable situation, it gives the "heads-up" to your body and you begin to do those things that you have the habit of doing when in an incongruent state.

The good news is that our bodies *also* do unconscious things when we are feeling amazing. Perhaps you smile more, whistle, play with your necklace or bop to music in your head.

To recognize your unfavourable behaviours, you need to become aware of how you move or behave just *before, during and after* an uncomfortable situation occurs. Once you've picked up on a few of them, try to recognize them the next time they happen and treat them as a warning sign. Some people refer to knowing something before it happens as intuition, a gut feeling or having a sixth sense. You may also think of it as your body talking to you. If you listen, you can learn to hone your sixth sense.

As you regularly edit your day ahead, you learn to point shift by recognizing what situations in your day may trigger your uncomfortable behaviours and you edit them out in advance.

Let's go back to our office scenario as an example. You edit *in* that while walking over to speak to your boss, instead of nervously jingling the keys in your pocket, you're softly whistling your favourite tune. Why? Because this is something you've noticed you do when you're feeling happy.

The Closer
The functional meditation closer, like the opener, is best accomplished by creating a mantra. Try something simple like "I'm entirely worthy of the ideal experience that I've created for myself. I deserve to be happy. I love myself enough to prove that I can achieve what I set out to accomplish. All that I do today will honour my life agenda."

Memorize the mantra you eventually settle on. It will confirm to you that you've created your day the way you want it to be and will be a fitting end to your daily practice.

Practice Makes Perfect
At first this is likely going to take you more like twenty minutes than five minutes. I actually hand out a chart to my patients, called "My Day Ahead," divided into three blank columns under

the headings "How I expect my next twenty-four hours to go," "The way I'd rather they go" and "Outcome." I encourage them to practise by taking some time before bed to think about and then fill in the chart. More often than not, when you reflect on your day in the Outcome column, things will have turned out the way you wished them to be, rather than the way you expected them to be. Such regular "proof" will keep you practising functional meditation. In fact, the more you practise, the more powerful the technique becomes and the less effort you'll expend (less effort equals less stress equals less free radicals).

Apply the twenty-one-day rule to this exercise and commit to the practice of functional meditation for at least three straight weeks. If you can do it for that long, chances are it will become a routine that will significantly reduce the stress in your life.

I've spent the last few pages outlining the practice of Functional Meditation, the technique I use to relieve the daily free radical load that results from stress. You may find other practices more suitable to your life and temperament. Just remember that you need to take action in some form to reduce your stress. Stress, as we saw earlier, is a major contributor to the body's oxidative burden. The ultimate goal is to relieve our bodies of as much disease risk as possible and to increase that buffer zone between our present health status and our personal health threshold.

—

CHAPTER 9

YOUR PERSONAL ANTIOXIDANT
NUTRITIONAL PLAN

After our childhood visits to our family doctor, who, as I mentioned in Chapter One, was a chiropractor, homeopath and naturopath rolled into one, my sisters and I looked forward with great excitement to our expedition to the local health food store near his office. Foods for Life was a shop in Toronto's Bloor West Village crammed with the latest in organic groceries, supplements and snacks.

"Right!" my mother would exclaim. "As a treat today, you each have a choice between organic yogurt-covered raisins, sesame snaps or a lovely carob bar that's completely free of sugar and bad fats!"

We'd jump and skip all the way to Foods for Life, ignoring the Baskin-Robbins ice cream store *at the very same corner*. My mother was a woman who was far ahead of her times, and she gave me a healthy grounding that made the path to healthy eating way less difficult for me to follow as I grew up than the nutritional grounding most of us are giving our children.

In this chapter, I'm going to set out a nutritional routine designed to get as much antioxidant power from your diet as possible. The word "diet" refers to whatever we eat, but in everyday speech, when we talk about "a diet," we're usually talking about some sort of caloric restriction. The antioxidant diet I'm going to present to you in this chapter is a diet in the first sense of the word—dynamic and subject to change. There's no fasting, starving or calorie counting here. But if you follow this antioxidant diet, you'll maintain an ideal weight, a lean body-mass ratio, an alert and balanced immune system and you'll literally wash your genes with nutritional information that will allow you to function with high energy, prevent disease onset and achieve optimal wellness.

In 2004, Franco and colleagues published a study in the *British Medical Journal* showing that an evidence-based way of eating—combining a lot of heart-friendly substances into something they called a "polymeal," which included wine, fish, dark chocolate, fruits, vegetables, almonds and garlic—was safer, cheaper, tastier and possibly more effective than the "polypill" method of treating heart disease with blood pressure medication, statins, water pills and Aspirins. Eating according to the polymeal plan reduced cardiovascular disease by 76 per cent in the study group. Following the plan, a male would perhaps increase his life expectancy by 6.6 years and thwart the onset of heart disease by 9 years; the corresponding statistics for women were 4.8 and 8.1 years respectively. The researchers concluded that the polymeal was an effective, non-pharmacological, safe, cheap and tasty alternative that would reduce cardiovascular morbidity and increase life expectancy.

The polymeal relies too heavily on the limited number of foods it recommends, but nevertheless it was one of my inspirations for the antioxidant nutrition plan I'm about to describe: one that is more complete, up-to-date and better designed than the polymeal. Free radicals and the antioxidant solution may be new science to us, but nature has always acknowledged this phenomenon, providing us with many natural antioxidants. They're right there in our food—the right food, that is. Through the study of antioxidants and nutrition, we know that food carries far more than just calories, vitamins and minerals. Many fruits and vegetables have immune-enhancing bioflavonoids, anti-inflammatory constituents and strong cancer-fighting properties. We'll be looking at which foods pack the most bang for your buck, but remember that even with the best antioxidant diet plan, changing your diet alone may not be enough to protect you. You will likely need the extra help of a personal antioxidant supplement plan—the subject of the next chapter.

Nutritional science has advanced beyond the familiar advice to avoid too many saturated fats, get lots of fibre, maintain a good level of hydration, keep sugar low and eat more fruits and vegetables. Studies at the United States Department of Agriculture and the Human Nutrition Research Center on Aging at Tufts University in Boston suggest that consuming fruits and vegetables with a high antioxidant value may help slow the aging process in both body and brain. Many other research projects now underway also suggest we should eat foods that have the highest *oxygen radical absorbance capacity* (ORAC—an acronym we'll be using a lot in this chapter). According to the latest scientific consensus, our best nutritional routine is based on foods that have the strongest antioxidant power; have beneficial, gene-modifying capacity; lower inflammation; enhance immune responses in the body; detoxify free radicals and prevent the onset of disease. ORAC foods are therapeutic foods as opposed to simply nutritionally fulfilling foods.

Oxygen radical absorption capacity is a helpful concept when we want to understand *which* foods have the highest antioxidant power. Don't confuse this with the measuring of free radical levels in our *bodies*, which we looked at in Chapter Five on testing. The ORAC value measures food's ability to give us what we need to reduce those free radicals.

As a rule of thumb, vibrantly coloured fruits and vegetables—red, orange, yellow and purple—contain the highest amounts of antioxidants. But they're far from the only sources. Chocolate, red wine and coffee are loaded with these radical fighters—though we need to consume such foods in moderation because, needless to say, a diet high in fat, alcohol or caffeine presents risks of other sorts. But we also don't want to miss their antioxidant benefits entirely and we certainly want to pay our respects to the "Come on! Live a little!" principle.

Consider the "French Paradox"—the low incidence of heart disease among a Mediterranean population that consumes fatty foods such as red meat and cheeses along with regular amounts of red wine and coffee—and the scientific evidence that blood serum antioxidant activity is higher in healthy volunteers who drink red wine than in those who do not. I think we can expect to see the ORAC label begin to appear on everything from packaged foods to herbs, supplements, candy bars and even bottles of wine.

In July 2006, a collaboration of Norwegian and U.S. scientists led by Nebte Halvorsen produced the largest ranking of antioxidant foods to date: over a thousand foods were studied, including processed foods and fresh fruits and vegetables. Blackberries are at the top of their list, with an antioxidant content of 5.75 millimoles per serving (millimoles are a measure of the amount of electrons/hydrogen atoms). The other antioxidant foods that make their top ten are walnuts, strawberries, artichokes, cranberries, coffee, raspberries, pecans, blueberries and ground cloves.

THE ORAC SUPERHEROES

All foods have an ORAC value. As we adapt to this new knowledge, we shouldn't purchase a food simply because its ORAC value is listed on the package. We need to know whether it really has a high ORAC value. Over time, you'll gain the experience you'll need to evaluate foods for their ORAC value by comparing them with what I like to call the ORAC superheroes. Right now, we commonly make such comparisons as, "That piece of cake has the fat content of a hamburger" or "That can of pop has the sugar value of two candy bars." Eventually we'll hear people saying, "That cereal has the ORAC value of half a cup of blueberries" or "That sauce has the ORAC value of a glass of red wine." Fat, sugar and carbohydrate content are all important to acknowledge, of course, but once we accept that the most important consideration is ORAC value, our diet will improve drastically.

If starting today you were to choose your grocery list on the basis of ORAC value, you'd have an outstanding diet, remain healthy and stay within your desired weight range.

You can probably even picture the list: fruits, vegetables, beans, grains, nuts and seeds, with lots of bright colours and variety. It may sound like your average "good food" list, but it's much more exciting than that. We're talking about berries and wine, tomatoes and garlic, coffee and chocolate, millet and quinoa, walnuts and pecans and lots of all-natural organic drinks and spices that are the ORAC superheroes. Let's get acquainted with them.

Fruits: Berries and Red Grapes

Okay, we all know fruits are healthy for us. They provide energy at a slower rate than pure sugar, are packed with vitamins and fibre, and beyond that, they're so tasty junk food manufacturers try to imitate them. But as with all foods, the ORAC value of fruit is of prime importance. Although almost all fruit has a respectable

ORAC value, the superheroes are berries and grapes. Don't let the fragile texture and easy spoiling of a berry fool you. In the world of ORAC value they are at the top of the list. Few fruits have the delightfully delicate allure or the nutrients of berries. Loaded with free radical scavengers, blueberries, raspberries and blackberries are rich in a special class of antioxidant called procyanidins that can help prevent cancer and heart disease and seem to be able to delay the onset of age-related loss of cognitive function. Strawberries, raspberries and blackberries also contain *ellagic acid,* a plant compound that combats carcinogens.

Red Wine

This is probably my favourite piece of advice in this entire book. One glass of red wine (preferably Cabernet because of the higher ORAC value and the procyanidin content) per day for women and two for men is ideal. By glass, I mean no more than 150 to 300 mL (5 to 10 ounces). Lots of studies suggest that red wine can keep you smarter, maintain a healthy and strong heart and protect your blood vessels from plaque development. The potent antioxidant substances resveratrol and quercetin, found in red grapes, also protect your heart against damaging free radicals. But the amount of resveratrol in red wine isn't enough; to reap resveratrol's benefits, you'll need the supplement form.

Red wine offers many other health benefits, including a reduction in platelet aggregation (blood stickiness) and an improvement in vasodilatory function that helps our blood vessels to remain open and flexible all the way to our brain. Resveratrol in the high amounts found in supplements can protect against cancer and reduce the risk of inflammatory diseases, gastric ulcers, stroke and even osteoporosis. The antioxidant value of red grape juice in its pure form is *nearly* as good for you as red wine.

The trouble with red wine is that many people are reluctant to stop drinking at one or two glasses. Unfortunately, more than the recommended amounts result in the *creation* of free radicals, not protection from them. Damage to your liver and arteries is the result.

Vegetables

I think perhaps just the memory of our moms pleading with us to eat our broccoli might have been enough to turn some of us off for life. But it's time to set childish things aside.

Broccoli

Broccoli and other Brassica *vegetables* such as kale, cabbage, rapini and Brussels sprouts can help prevent cancer and ward off heart disease. Also known as cruciferous vegetables, this group contains a compound called *indole-3-carbinol* (I3C)—a potent antioxidant that breaks down estrogen in the body. The compound I3C reduces the risk of breast cancer and other estrogen-sensitive cancers such as cancer of the ovaries and cervix. These vegetables contain other protective antioxidants such as beta-carotene, which also helps prevent cancer and heart disease. Studies have shown that broccoli can help fight cervical dysplasia, a precancerous condition. There is much talk these days about immunization against cervical dysplasia that is caused by the human papilloma virus (HPV). I favour a daily plate of broccoli, kale and mustard greens rather than adding yet another vaccine to the ever-growing list administered to our preteen population.

Spinach

Spinach doesn't just give Popeye stronger forearms; it offers significant protection for our vision. Lutein is the antioxidant found in spinach and a crucial nutrient for the health of the human eye.

Studies have demonstrated that people who eat spinach are less likely to develop cataracts and macular degeneration. Lutein protects your retina (the visual receptor at the back of the eye) from sunlight-caused free radicals.

Garlic

Some call garlic a panacea or cure-all because it is one of the world's oldest known medicinal herbs. A sulphur compound is responsible for both garlic's pungent odour and the healing benefits. Garlic is packed with antioxidants to help fend off cancer, heart disease and the effects of aging. It fights free radicals, lowers cholesterol, works to reduce blood pressure and keeps our blood from clotting. Besides warding off Dracula and keeping the ticker healthy, garlic's efficacy in treating yeast infections is well known.

Tomatoes

Regular consumption of tomatoes has been associated with decreased risk of chronic degenerative diseases. Tomatoes contain the antioxidant *lycopene*, which we'll be looking at further in our supplement chapter. It's actually more powerful than beta-carotene or glutathione, which boosts immune and liver function. Those with sensitivities to the nightshade family of vegetables have to be careful with tomatoes, potatoes, bell peppers, chilies and cayenne pepper, and eggplant because these foods can contribute to arthritis and some other inflammatory diseases. But for most of us, tomatoes are on the list of superhero foods for good reason: they can ward off certain kinds of cancer. They're especially well known for their protection of the prostate gland. Recent studies have shown that men who eat the equivalent of one can of tomato paste daily have significantly lower rates of prostate cancer. Other studies have suggested that lycopene may help prevent lung, colon and breast cancers. Tomatoes also protect the eyes against macular degeneration and cataracts, and support mental function and successful aging.

People generally assume that eating vegetables raw is always best. In fact, this depends on the vegetable. Heating tomatoes allows more desirable antioxidants to be available to the body, making tomato sauce the best way to consume them. Cooking also lowers the acidity level.

Carrots

I have to be honest, carrots come last on my list of veggies because they're already well admired. They're sweet and crunchy, a favourite snack loaded with a potent antioxidant called beta-carotene (a precursor to vitamin A). I have no problem persuading health-conscious people to eat more of them. But be careful about eating too many; they pack a sugar wallop and are high on the glycemic index (GI). (This index ranks carbohydrates based on their effects on glucose levels in the blood. Carbohydrates with lower GI ratings are digested more slowly, with the result that more nutrition is extracted from them, lower insulin levels are required and less sugar finds its way to the blood. This in turn keeps inflammation potential low, lowering the overall amount of circulating free radicals.)

High levels of beta-carotene can also be found in beets, sweet potatoes and winter squash (all of which are also high GI veggies). Beta-carotene and the other carotenoids have been carefully studied and certainly do provide protection against cancer and heart disease and can help in the treatment of arthritis. Just like tomatoes, cooking carrots by lightly steaming them or including them in a pasta sauce or soup helps the body access their carotenoid antioxidants.

The Humble Seed

These include beans, grains, nuts, seeds and legumes—those little kernels of life that so often fail to get the acclaim they deserve. I could easily put seeds at the top of the ORAC list—soybeans and small red beans are both antioxidant superheroes. But do you realize that these country cousins have city cousins that are delicious and exciting? And here's the shocker: delicious and exciting doesn't mean bad for you. So I'm going to start with a wonderful food that, most of the time, we hardly remember was once a bean.

Chocolate: The Luscious Bean

The cacao "bean" is the seed of the cacao tree, a native of South America. The bean itself is bitter, but when processed as chocolate, the result is delicious. Research has demonstrated that the antioxidants in cacao are exceptionally easily absorbed and ever so useful to our body. Cornell University food scientists found that cocoa powder has nearly twice the antioxidants of red wine and up to three times what is found in green tea. Since I reviewed this research a few years back, a night rarely goes by that I don't have a glass of red wine with a velvety piece of chocolate with 90 per cent cacao content.

The findings were published in an article entitled "Cocoa Has More Phenolic Phytochemicals and a Higher Antioxidant Capacity than Teas and Red Wine" in the American Chemical Society's *Journal of Agriculture and Food Chemistry*. The Cornell University researchers who authored the paper showed chocolate to have a high content of antioxidant compounds called *phenolic phytochemicals*, or *flavonoids*. They discovered huge amounts of antioxidants in a single serving of cocoa. But don't start including average milk chocolate in your diet. Chocolate manufacturers have worked for decades to *remove* the bitter antioxidants and create a candy taste by adding milk and cream for smoothness and a whack of sugar for sweetness. The result, I'm afraid, is a food item that *causes* heart disease and free radicals instead of protecting us from them. My prescription is two small squares a day of a dark chocolate containing 70 per cent or more cacao. This kind of chocolate, like coffee, is deliciously bitter. For some people, the taste is acquired, but it's worth acquiring for reasons of both health and pleasure.

Coffee: The Magic Bean

Many natural health practitioners advocate no coffee, but in my opinion this advice is wrong. Coffee has received some negative press in the past, primarily because of its well-known jangly effects when taken to excess. But coffee in small amounts is very good for you. Beyond adding a jolt of mental alertness, coffee has a significant antioxidant effect, and may have an inverse association with the risk of type 2 diabetes mellitus. Other research suggests that people from families prone to Parkinson's disease who drink coffee are less likely to develop the disease. This is a further clue as to how environment works with genes to cause disease—the genomics factor discussed in Chapter Four. Dr. William Scott of the University of Miami School of Medicine, who has carried out some of the most important research in this area, suggests that the findings point clearly to *dopamine*, one of the feel-good chemicals in the brain, which falls to low levels in Parkinson's sufferers. The researchers can't yet say with certainty what mechanism can be attributed to coffee. I suspect the positive effects will be traced to antioxidant protection, since Parkinson's disease is caused when the brain cells that produce dopamine die, largely as a result of attack by free radicals, in some cases caused by pesticides that are known to be strongly linked with disease risk.

The disease is progressive, affecting about 1 per cent of people older than sixty-five.

Coffee's protective antioxidant effects are good news for coffee lovers, especially because, besides enhancing blood flow to the head, some studies have linked its consumption to possible protection against liver and colon cancer as well as type 2 diabetes. According to a study by researchers at the University of Scranton, Pennsylvania, Americans get more of their antioxidants from coffee than any other dietary source. It would be much better if we got our antioxidants from fruits and vegetables. Although coffee is an antioxidant superhero, it is not the caffeine that adds the antioxidant properties. Decaf delivers them in full measure but avoids the potential elevation in blood pressure and other unwanted side effects from the standard cup o' joe.

I strongly recommend one daily cup of black, organic coffee—a half-and-half mixture of Swiss water-decaffeinated beans and caffeinated—best consumed before noon. If you're not a coffee drinker to begin with and don't really like the taste, try organic decaf green tea instead.

Soybeans

The well-studied health benefits of soy, for women and men, stem from its phytoestrogens—natural plant estrogens that resemble estrogens in the body but are weaker and help *prevent* cancer. A family of phytoestrogens called isoflavones includes a compound called *genistein*, also found in soy. Isoflavones help to prevent cancer, lower cholesterol, ward off osteoporosis and lessen the effects of menopause; studies have shown that genistein can help prevent breast, colon and prostate cancers. Soy can also reduce overall cholesterol levels and the levels of low-density lipoprotein (LDL or "bad" cholesterol) levels, without affecting "good" cholesterol, HDL. Soy can also prevent osteoporosis and help alleviate the symptoms of menopause.

Small Red Beans

These are not quite as popular as coffee and chocolate, nor as well studied as the berry fruits, but small red beans have incredible ORAC value. The lesson here is: don't judge a food's antioxidant power by its aesthetic or taste appeal. Red beans look like kidney beans. They are the same colour and shape except that the red bean is slightly smaller. It is also known as the Mexican red bean, but is grown in many parts of North America. Although red beans come near the top of the ORAC list, we don't need to eat bowls of dried small red beans every day—that might lose us friends! Instead, remember to mix them into salads, sauces, soups, and baked goods (beans in baked goods add great texture and nutritional value and don't affect the flavour of the recipe). We need to eat a wide variety of antioxidant-rich foods to ensure an adequate intake of all nutrients.

Whole Grains

Grains are seeds too, and wheat isn't the only grain on the planet. Millet, quinoa, kasha and amaranth grains are creating a revolution in our food tastes. Our morning bowl of cereal is a potent source of phytochemicals as long as it's the whole-grain variety. "Whole grain" doesn't have to mean "whole wheat," nor does it necessarily mean a dark brown piece of bread. It means that we're cooking (often boiling) whole grains either on their own as a side dish or in combination for cereal, or perhaps mixing them into soups or making casseroles. The vitamin E in grains is a potent antioxidant that plays a role in preventing cancer, especially prostate cancer. Other studies have found that vitamin E can boost immunity, slow the progression of Alzheimer's disease, treat and possibly prevent arthritis, prevent sunburn and treat male infertility. Grains are also rich in *phytic acid*, known as IP-6, a potent antioxidant that can help protect against breast, colon and liver cancers. My recommendation is no less than two cups per day of high fibre, multinutritional, life-sustaining grains.

Nuts and Other Seeds

The recognition that omega-3 fatty acids were missing from our diets has gone mainstream. They are *necessary* nutrients, not true antioxidants, but omega-3 fish oil supplements often require antioxidants *in* them as preservatives to prevent them from going rancid. Omega-3s are found in fish, nuts, seeds, algae and certain animal products. Many studies have demonstrated that they're great for your heart and brain function. Nuts and seeds have recently gained in popularity because of their omega-3 content. But nuts and seeds have great antioxidant power as well, at least enough to make it onto my list of antioxidant superheroes, though perhaps by the skin of their teeth. Walnuts, pecans, hazelnuts and almonds top the nut list for their nutritional benefits and antioxidant power. Where seeds are concerned, I like the many benefits that sunflower, pumpkin and sesame seeds have to offer, including their high calcium and zinc content. I recommend no more but no less than the equivalent of one handful of fresh (non-rancid) unsalted, un-roasted nuts and seeds, five times a week.

Herbs and Spices

They're robust, tangy and pungent. They're perfect for soups and stews, accents on pizza, in cheese dips and even desserts—and now we learn they are good for us too. U.S. Department of Agriculture scientists recently carried out a study of twenty-seven culinary and twelve medicinal herbs that revealed that many popular herbs are a great source of natural antioxidants. In fact, the total phenolic content (the antioxidant ingredient) of many herbs in the study is higher than those reported for berries, fruits and vegetables. Although we would have to eat an awful lot of herbs to get the equivalent total amount of antioxidants we can consume in fruits and vegetables, supplementing an otherwise balanced diet with herbs appears to be highly beneficial to our health.

Tea

You may not think of it this way, but tea is among the world's most popular herbs. It may also be one of the best ways to prevent a number of degenerative diseases. Tea, the most frequently consumed beverage in the world, has been shown to significantly reduce the risk of cancer, heart disease, stroke and other diseases. It was originally thought that green tea had more antioxidants than black tea, but recent studies suggest that they're equally beneficial. Some late breaking news: squeeze half a lemon into your green tea (cold or hot) to increase and preserve the antioxidant effects of the tea's catechins (the antioxidant ingredient) and make them more easily absorbed by the body.

WHAT WE SHOULD EAT

The Chicago-based Institute of Food Technologists reported that sales of products carrying an antioxidant claim jumped nearly 20 per cent last year. One of every 4 consumers claims to eat fruits or vegetables to prevent disease, 1 in 3 eats them to feel healthy, and nearly 9 of 10 eat them to stay healthy. But we're still not eating enough of these disease-fighting foods. And there's no doubt we need more specific advice.

Though Canada is sometimes ahead of the United States in health-related issues, this is not true when it comes to nutrition. The new Canadian Food Guide teaches us that vegetables and fruits make up the largest arc of Canada's Food Guide "rainbow" and suggests that a healthy diet rich in a variety of vegetables and fruits may help reduce the risk of some types of cancer. This is true. It also suggests that eating lots of vegetables and fruits regularly may lower your risk of heart disease as well. This too is true. But it suggests that eating at least one serving of vegetables or fruits at every meal and as a snack provides us with the amount of vegetables and fruits we need each day. Assuming three meals per day and two snacks, that amounts to five servings a day.

But we now know that, as a result of the bombardment of toxins in our environment, our general lack of exercise and the overwhelming availability of fast food, *five servings fall far short of our requirements for optimal health.*

What are the requirements then? More than most of us consume, I'm afraid. If you don't count potatoes, the average person gets a total of just three servings of fruits and vegetables a day. Yet the latest dietary guidelines call for up to *thirteen* servings of fruits and vegetables a day. An average male, who needs about 2,000 calories a day to maintain his weight and health, requires a minimum of *nine* servings, or more than one litre (four *cups*) per day.

250 mL (1 cup) of fruit is equal to one of the following:

1 medium grapefruit

1 large banana

1 small apple

1 medium pear

1 small wedge of watermelon

1 large orange

3 medium plums

8 large strawberries

250 mL (1 cup) of vegetables/salad is equal to one of the following:

1 large bell pepper

2 large celery stalks

1 medium potato (preferably baked, not fried)

250 mL (1 cup) of cooked or 500 mL (2 cups) of raw greens

(spinach, collards, mustard greens, turnip greens)

1 large sweet potato

12 baby carrots (or 2 medium carrots)

250 mL (2 cups) 10 broccoli or cauliflower florets

1 cup of green beans

500 mL (2 cups) of lettuce (counts as 250 mL (1 cup) of vegetables)

If we attempt to follow the thirteen-servings-a-day recommendation, we must be careful. Thirteen servings of fruits and vegetables that include loads of nuts and berries may contain about 16,000 ORAC units. On the other hand, if these servings are mostly salads made from iceberg lettuce, which has little to no ORAC value, they may account for less than 500 ORAC units. Fresh fruits have on average about four times higher ORAC value than fresh vegetables. Everything depends on our choices.

FOODS WE SHOULD NOT EAT

The list of things we should eat is much shorter than the list of things we need to avoid.

Here's a worst-ten list.

1. *Fast food.* You don't need me to go into more detail about fast foods. Avoid 'em.
2. *Hydrogenated fats*, as we all know by now, *must* be avoided because they cause heart disease. They've been

used for years in snack foods, bakery items and margarine. Avoid buying cookies, crackers, baked goods or anything else that has hydrogenated oil or trans-fats on the ingredients list.

3. *Olestra* is a *synthetic* fat used to make non-fat potato chips and other snacks. You'd think, with all the bad rap fat has garnered, a non-fat fat would be great. But Olestra has been shown to bind with fat-soluble vitamins A, E, D and K and carotenoids—our invaluable antioxidant nutrients—and to eliminate them from the system. Never mind the fact that Olestra causes stomach upset and, er, other digestive problems, its consumption encourages people to skip over fruits and vegetables for snacks that appear to offer no threat.

4. *Nitrates*, found at high levels in cured meats such as bacon and hot dogs, preserve colour and prevent microbes from taking up residence. But they're bad— really bad. The *nitrate* itself is harmless, but it can convert to *nitrite* in your body, which in turn can form *nitrosamines*, powerful cancer-causing chemicals. Whenever possible, look for nitrate-free organic meats. If you must eat foods containing nitrates, take extra vitamin C as it is known to prevent the conversion to nitrosamines in your stomach.

5. *Alcohol*—I'm not talking here about moderate amounts of red wine—causes many problems. Liver toxicity is the main issue when we exceed our limits, and this, as we've learned, causes free radical excess.

6. *Raw oysters and sushi* are great but they can carry deadly bacteria that can cause severe illness or death. You take a big risk every time you consume them. To date, no government or independent body inspects seafood for safety

or will guarantee its quality. Oysters and fish are usually safe and nutritious foods if you cook them first.

7. *Saturated animal fats* include the fatty meats, especially beef and pork, or the skin on poultry. It also includes full-fat dairy products such as cheese, milk and cream. Fatty meat and dairy products do have some contributions to make to a diet—including nutrients that feed your brain—but not many that can't be found elsewhere.

8. *Soda pop* is a poor way to get fluids in the short term and a great way to develop diabetes in the longer term. Pop is full of sugar or artificial sweeteners and often contains caffeine, artificial colours and flavours. Replace pop by mixing sparkling water with fresh, pure juice. Bonus: the sparkling juice tastes better than pop. (That's why pop bottlers try to imitate it.)

9. *High-fat and high-sodium snacks*, including chips, even if they are made with vegetable oil. Try to avoid these. The balance of fat in our diets has shifted too far towards the omega-6 variety found in most processed vegetable oils. We way overdo salt, leading to many cases of high blood pressure. And there's now evidence that too many of these fats and sodium-rich foods may be leading to specific chronic diseases. One reason we want to supplement the diet with the necessary omega-3 oils is to regain the proper omega balance and prevent everything from inflammation to heart disease.

10. *Frozen meals* may not be inherently bad for you if they have all the "right" ingredients in them, but they do keep you from eating *fresh*, whole, natural foods that contain more nutrients and fibre and disease-fighting phyto-chemicals. You may be tempted to excuse them as "better than fast food." You may be sometimes pressured for

time. But don't let simple laziness displace real foods in *your* diet.

YOUR PERSONAL ANTIOXIDANT NUTRITION PLAN

I call our antioxidant routine a plan, not a diet, because "diets"—nutritional routines aimed specifically at weight loss—are usually unsuccessful and may even put your life at risk. The tragedy is that dieting has become a cultural or fashionable norm. Lots of people spend many years and much money dieting when there's no evidence to suggest that these diets result in any long-term weight loss or health benefits at all. You're going to lose the wrong type of weight on any conventional diet, because these diets cannot help but promote the loss of lean body mass. Some very compelling studies have shown that 95 per cent of all dieters regain their lost weight.

Dieters don't get enough calcium; experience loss of muscular mass, strength and endurance; have decreased oxygen utilization, thinning hair, loss of coordination, dehydration and electrolyte imbalances; and experience fainting, weakness and slowed heart rates. Dieting also affects the mind. When we restrict calories we restrict our energy, which in turn can restrict our brainpower. A conventional dieting effort puts our bodies into "starvation mode," which causes a significant degree of free radical accumulation as well as a deficiency of antioxidants—especially the fat-soluble A, E, D and K vitamins that are lost when the body's percentage of fat drops drastically during dieting.

The antioxidant nutrition plan I'm offering you is a set of rules for healthy eating. It requires only that you consume those foods highest in ORAC value. If you do, you'll lose the necessary weight at a healthy and sustainable rate (about 1 kg [2 lb.] per week) until you've reached your ideal body mass. You'll never have to diet in the sense of counting calories, feeling hungry, purchasing hard-to-find food laden with sugar-free chemicals or being "medically supervised." Not ever.

Our emphasis on foods of high ORAC value means you eat well—probably as well as human beings can possibly eat—and you won't be starving yourself, won't be depriving your body of vital nutrients and won't be setting yourself up for a compensating binge. Why binge to recover from a diet that includes chocolate, wine, meat and a boundless supply of vegetables of every sort? Of course, following the plan, you'll eat less than you did if you're someone who has habitually overindulged. But you won't feel deprived of the sheer fun of good food. With the supplement plan and the exercise routine we're going to look at in the next chapters, our antioxidant nutrition plan is all you need to achieve optimal health.

Getting Started

I'd like you to record the quantity of everything you eat and drink for two weeks, including the times of day for each meal or snack. Writing stuff down prevents the distortions of memory. Don't start the program or alter your habits until you review them two weeks after you've begun this journal. This is for your sake. I want you to be able to compare what you now eat in a typical week with what the plan recommends. At the end of two weeks, you can make the comparison and begin to shape your strategy.

The rules for the plan are below. Be patient with yourself. Not many of us can follow every rule from the outset. If your two-week study of your habits suggests that you're going to experience a lot of trouble, say, getting the necessary daily servings of vegetables, you can try preparing them in advance. Chop a variety of veggies, say, enough to fill a huge glass container. Then, as you need them, take three or four servings with you to work. Eat some in the car, some on break and some on the way home. Easy.

Reevaluate yourself after one month. Repeat this reevaluation procedure until you find that you have incorporated all the rules into your daily nutritional routine.

Relish your success as a non-dieter.

THE RULES FOR YOUR ANTIOXIDANT NUTRITION PLAN

The secret of my nutrition plan is that you'll turn it into a way of life simply because *you'll feel so good*. You may have to exercise some willpower, yet remain balanced and never become fanatical.

1. **QUALITY:** Assure that every item of food you eat has the highest possible antioxidant (ORAC) value within its group and class. Cross-check the "grocery list" that I provide for you below. Your diet is going to include a lot of beans, berries, colourful fruits and vegetables—at least seven servings a day—and that 70 per cent chocolate and even one or two glasses of red wine.

   If it doesn't originate in nature, or it isn't organic, or it's sprayed with pesticides, don't touch it. Pesticides, as we've learned, wreak havoc on the nervous system by way of free radicals. Purchase only foods labelled "certified organic."

2. **METHOD:** Chew your food until it is liquefied before you swallow it. Use digestive enzymes with larger meals if you currently experience indigestion, heartburn, gas or bloating. Digestive enzymes can help ensure that you absorb everything you ingest. Remember, you are what you eat, but more importantly, you are what you *absorb*. I would recommend a broad-spectrum enzyme that you

can take in capsule form. These supplements are high in plant-based protease, lipase and amylase enzymes.

3. **TIMING:** Don't skip meals. Listen to your body and eat when you're slightly hungry, not starving. Aim for six meals a day (three main meals, two snacks, and a couple of squares of 70 per cent chocolate in the evening). If you use nutrition bars or shakes, use only the well-formulated ones that provide less than 300 calories, with less than 15 per cent of these calories coming from carbohydrates (including sugars) and at least 40 per cent of the calories coming from protein. Consume such snacks *between* meals only, and don't forget to avoid the ones with preservatives and artificial colours.

4. **PREPARATION:** For convenience, prepare some of your staple foods in bulk in advance. Don't hesitate to preboil grains, precut fruits and vegetables and grill your meat in advance. Use glass containers to freeze and to prepackage this food. Avoid storing food in plastic. Avoid microwaving, frying and barbecuing. Instead, grill, steam, broil and boil, methods that cause less free radical damage to the food.

5. **QUANTITY:** Try eating meals from small "dessert" plates. Listen to your body for signs of moderate hunger or low blood sugar. You know you've waited too long to eat when you start getting shaky, becoming forgetful, irritable or light-headed. Earn your food by remaining active, but don't focus on exact amounts or calorie counting. Wait at least thirty minutes from the time you've started your first helping before you think about having seconds. It takes a minimum of ten to fifteen minutes to eat the amount of food on your plate and then about fifteen minutes for your brain to register the satisfaction of having eaten this food.

6. **HYDRATION:** Drink lots of water, but make sure to drink most of it between meals so as not to dilute your digestive enzymes during mealtime.

7. **WHAT NOT TO EAT:** This rule is a variation on the Remove principle we talked about as one of the four Rs. It is also highlighted in my "worst-ten" foods list above. When you remove harmful and oxidizing foods from your diet, you make the task of combatting free radicals that much easier.

   Beyond those baddies you'll avoid outright, you'll also want to seriously limit the following:

   - Fat. When you do require fat, use olive oil or a very small amount of butter.
   - Sugar (or its equivalents such as brown sugar, syrup, honey or molasses). Try using stevia or moderate amounts of agave nectar as a replacement sweetener.
   - Refined carbohydrates such as pasta, bread, cakes, cookies.
   - Not more than one serving of wheat-based products a day.
   - Not more than one serving of dairy products a day.
   - No alcohol except for the recommended wine.
   - Not more than one serving of red meat a week.

8. **NEVER PLAN A CHEAT DAY:** Birthdays, weddings, holidays and other special occasions for eating happen as often as once per week for many of us. My rule is that when these celebrations occur, ignore the no-go foods, have fun and enjoy *in moderation*. But when special occasions occur more than once a week, it's carrot sticks for you, not birthday cake.

The Calorie Concept

Again, this nutritional plan is not a diet. Women tend to picture an ideal weight that is unrealistically low, so they're more likely to diet unnecessarily. Men tend to imagine their ideal weight to be higher than medically recommended. We are not "dieting" here in the usual sense, so we won't dwell on calories or weight, but it's sensible to have a clear idea of your energy requirements.

Studies done on slowing the aging process suggest that we should aim to consume slightly—about 200 calories—under our caloric demands in order to keep free radicals under control. Other experts suggest this may add years to your life expectancy, at the cost of being chronically hungry with a gurgling stomach for all those extra years. In the section "A Daily Menu" below, I've used an example of a person requiring 1,800 calories a day. To calculate your approximate caloric needs, try using this simple formula.

Desired (ideal) weight (in pounds) x 10 = calories needed
(Add approximately 200 extra calories on days you exercise.)

Your desired or ideal weight must take into account the composition of your body: how much of your weight is lean body mass (muscle and bone) and how much is body fat. For optimum health, your body fat should be no more than 20 per cent of your total body weight for men and no more than 30 per cent for women. Of course you can't determine this by standing on a bathroom scale. But look for a practitioner who has a new model body impedance analysis (BIA) device that measures full body composition. BIA has come into favour in recent years because it can accurately measure body fat, total body water and fat-free body mass (lean tissue and muscle mass).

I won't say much more about the limited value of comparing calories. But consider this. Three large antioxidant-rich apples (385 g [13.5 oz.]), three slices of free radical-rich bacon (34 g [1.2 oz.]), eight large free radical-fighting kiwis (328 g [12 oz.]) and one pad of strongly oxidizing butter (28 g [1 oz.]) are equivalent to 200 calories each. The message is clear: high-powered antioxidant foods are also those that are lower in calories overall. It's no coincidence that antioxidant foods are also the healthiest foods known—the highest in fibre, the lowest in fat and the most truly able to prevent disease.

Try not to get stuck in the routine of eating the same foods every single day as a matter of convenience. Whether or not foods are high ORAC, they must be rotated to ensure a healthy immune system and to avoid food intolerances and sensitivities. That means that it might even be a good idea to switch your favourite wine and coffee on a regular basis, while always keeping it organic.

The Shopping List

Now let's go shopping for antioxidant foods you can rely on while you're setting up your plan. What we're aiming at here is a lifelong routine, not some three-week wonder. Of course I'm not suggesting that you can never have any food that *isn't* on this list. But I've compiled this "best-of-the-best" list for you by looking at the antioxidant power of more than a thousand foods and consulting five major studies on ORAC value. You'll be rewarded by the greatest benefits if you stick closely to these recommendations most of the time.

Within each grouping, I've listed the foods from highest to lowest antioxidant (ORAC) value. In addition to the potent ingredients called phytonutrients that consistently place the fruits and vegetables in first ORAC position, all these foods have great

ORAC values because they carry formidable amounts of vitamins A, C and E and selenium—the ACES. Before we get to the shopping list, let's just use this table to underline the foods that pack these important nutrients.

WHO'S HOLDING THE ACES?	
Antioxidant	**Good Food Sources**
Beta-carotene (vitamin A)	Dark orange, red, yellow and green vegetables and fruits such as broccoli, kale, spinach, sweet potatoes, carrots, red and yellow peppers, apricots, cantaloupe and mangos.
Vitamin C	Berries, dark green vegetables (spinach, asparagus, green peppers, Brussels sprouts, broccoli, watercress, other greens), red and yellow peppers, tomatoes and tomato juice, mangos, papaya and guava.
Vitamin E	Vegetable oils such as olive, soybean oil, nuts and nut butters, seeds, whole grains, wheat, wheat germ, brown rice, oatmeal, soybeans, sweet potatoes, legumes (beans, lentils, split peas) and dark green leafy vegetables.
Selenium	Brazil nuts, brewer's yeast, oatmeal, brown rice, chicken, eggs, dairy products, garlic, molasses, onions, salmon, seafood, tuna, wheat germ, whole grains, most vegetables.

The ratings I assign to foods are based on their total antioxidant value. This shopping list is firmly based in good science. You'll see right away that this list is drawn from our catalogue of antioxidant superheroes. The foods are all measured in millimoles per 100 mg—the amount of electrons/hydrogen atoms donated by a 100 g sample of the food—in other words, *their ability to act as antioxidants.*

Antioxidant power isn't the only basis for appearing on our shopping list. Anti-inflammatory characteristics (though I suggest caution in respect to nightshade vegetables and citrus fruits) are also important, as is a great—that is, low—glycemic index. Foods with a low glycemic index don't cause the inflammation that typically invites free radical damage. So all of these factors work nicely together.

THE ANTIOXIDANT SHOPPING LIST

Category 1: FRUITS (raw)	ORAC Value (mmol/100 g)
Elderberry	14.70
Cranberry	9.58
Plum	7.58
Blueberry	6.55
Prune	6.55
Blackberry	5.35
Raspberry	4.88
Apple (Red Delicious)	4.27
Apple (Granny Smith)	3.90
Strawberry	3.58
Cherry	3.36
Gooseberry	3.27
Pear	2.94
Avocado	1.93
Orange (navel)	1.82
Tangerine	1.62
Grapefruit	1.55
Grape (red)	1.26
Apricot	1.11
Mango	1.00
Kiwi	0.88

Category 2: VEGETABLES	ORAC Value (mmol/100 g)
(Make them steamed and always try to add spices for enhanced ORAC value and flavour!)	
Artichoke (steamed)	9.41
Red cabbage (steamed)	3.14
Rapini or broccoli rabb (raw)	3.08
†Russet potato (baked)	1.68
Spinach	1.5
Butternut squash	0.39
†Red bell peppers	0.79

Category 3: GRAINS
(Note: Any time you mix grains and beans together, you get all of the twenty amino acids necessary for health—without having to eat meat!)

Oats (uncooked)	1.71
Amaranth	N/A
Barley	N/A
Brown rice	N/A
Buckwheat	N/A

N/A = not applicable (these foods have either a very strong anti-inflammatory value or an ORAC value yet to be determined, or both).
†Nightshade vegetables, which could possibly be pro-inflammatory in some people.
Orac values based on the 2007 list prepared by the Nutrient Data Labratory, Beltsville Nutrition Research Center, Agricultural Research Service and the U.S. Department of Agriculture and the 2006 list prepared by Halvorsen et al.

Category 3: GRAINS (cont'd)	ORAC Value (mmol/100g)
Millet	N/A
Quinoa	N/A
Rye	N/A

Category 4: BEANS (Legumes)
(Note: Any time you mix grains and beans together, you get all of the twenty amino acids necessary for health—without having to eat meat!)

Small red beans	14.92
Red kidney beans	8.46
Black beans	8.04
Pinto beans	7.77
Lentils	7.28
Soybeans (and tofu)	5.76
Black-eyed peas	4.34
Cashews	1.94
Navy beans	1.52
Chick peas	0.85
Split peas	0.52
Adzuki beans	N/A
Broad beans	N/A
Mung beans	N/A

Category 5: NUTS AND SEEDS
(Note: Avoid old, rancid, salted or roasted nuts. You may choose to lightly roast and salt on your own, but nuts sold this way may be hiding their oxidized taste.)

Pecans	17.94
Walnuts	13.54
Hazelnuts	9.64
Pistachios	7.98
Almonds	4.45
Macadamia nuts	1.69
Brazil nuts	1.42
Flaxseed (ground)	1.12
Pumpkin seed	N/A
Soy nuts	N/A
Sunflower seeds	N/A

Category 6: MEAT AND FISH	ORAC Value (mmol/100 g)

(Note: Almost all animal product is low ORAC, but when lean and organic it can provide great nutrition.)

Fish
(Note: Baked or broiled.)

Tilapia	0.14
Tuna (canned)	0.12
Salmon (canned)	0.10
Cod	N/A
Halibut	N/A
Mackerel	N/A
Sardines	N/A

POULTRY
Chicken

(White meat, organic, free-range whenever possible, boneless, skinless, prepared baked or broiled.)	N/A

Turkey

(White meat, organic and free-range whenever possible, prepared baked or broiled.)	N/A

Category 7: OILS
(for cooking and on salads)

Olive oil (extra virgin)	1.15

Category 8: DAIRY
(These are the only dairy products I include, since others have pro-inflammatory potential.)

Yogurt (1%)	0.04
Whole egg	0.04
Organic skim milk	N/A
Pecorino cheese	N/A

Category 9: HERBS AND SPICES	ORAC Value (mmol/100 g)
Cloves	314.46
Cinnamon	267.53
Oregano	200.13
Parsley	74.35
Basil	67.55
Curry	48.50
Sage (fresh)	32.00
Mustard (seed)	29.25
Black pepper	27.62
Thyme (fresh)	27.42
Chili	23.64
Ginger	21.57
Paprika	17.92
Turmeric	15.68
Garlic	6.66
Coriander (fresh)	5.14
Dill (fresh)	4.39
Cardamom	2.76
Bay leaf	N/A
Rosemary	N/A

Category 10: SWEETENERS (Note: Use in moderation.)	ORAC Value (mmol/100 g)
Molasses (dark and blackstrap)	4.90
Barley malt syrup (organic)	2.12

OTHER

	ORAC Value (mmol/100 g)
Chocolate (dark, minimum 70% cacao)	20.82

Drinks

Red wine (Cabernet Sauvignon)	5.03
Coffee	1.25
Grape juice	1.01
Water	

(Water has no ORAC value, of course, but you need to stay well hydrated.)

A DAILY MENU

Here's a typical daily menu from the antioxidant nutrition plan, representing an intake of 1,800 calories a day. But remember that you need only approximate your caloric demands (see the formula on page 153) and follow the eight rules. The quantity you eat will turn out just fine.

On waking:
500 mL (17 oz.) of room-temperature water with lemon. Detoxifying!

Breakfast: (with suggested amounts of vitamins and antioxidants as outlined in Chapter Ten, "Your Personal Antioxidant Supplement Plan")

1 small organic black coffee, if desired
2 selections from Fruits (preferably berries)
1 selection from Vegetables
1 selection each from Grains, Beans, and Nuts and Seeds or 1 selection from Meat or 1 selection from Dairy
500 mL (17 oz.) water

Snack:
2 selections from Fruits

Lunch:
2 selections from Vegetables
1 selection each from Grains and Beans or 1 selection from Meat
500 mL (17 oz.) water

Snack:
2 selections from Vegetables and 1 selection from Nuts and Seeds
500 mL (17 oz.) water

Dinner: (with suggested amounts of vitamins and antioxidants outlined in Chapter Ten, "Your Personal Antioxidant Supplement Plan")

Salad—at least 3 selections (including lettuce) from Vegetables
1 selection from Grains, Beans (Legumes)
1 selection from Meat
Organic red wine. Women: 1 glass. Men: 2 glasses
500 mL (17 oz.) water

Snack:
2 squares of unsweetened minimum 70% cacao chocolate (optional)

This isn't an onerous diet of deprivation. It's a flexible menu of delicious foods that all have one crucial characteristic: they're powerful antioxidants.

COOKING METHODS

Despite a lingering notion that raw foods are preferable to cooked ones, steaming and broiling food has been shown to yield slightly higher levels of antioxidants than eating food raw. Frying in oil introduces more fat into our diet. People who have unthinkingly accepted the view that frying makes everything taste better are often surprised to discover the delights of broiled and roasted vegetables.

As to the preparation of food in microwave ovens, I'm afraid the jury is still out. We may not have seen any reliable studies suggesting that microwaving food leads to cancer, but there is now strong evidence that microwave cooking creates a lower antioxidant value in your food.

The notion that cooking methods—and even cookware—may play a role in free radical creation has gained currency in the market. A stainless steel set of cookware is now available that incorporates a battery-powered unit in the handle of each pot and pan that is designed to generate an electrical charge that is said to minimize the free radicals created during the cooking process by supplying missing electrons to these radicals as they're created.

FOOD INTOLERANCE

A serious problem with modern diets, one that indirectly contributes to free radical burden, is food sensitivity, also known as food intolerance. Symptoms of food intolerance are numerous and can include acne, anxiety, arthritis, asthma, attention deficit disorder, autism, chronic diarrhea, chronic fatigue, constipation, depression, diabetes, eczema, headaches (tension type and migraine), high blood pressure, hyperactivity disorder, irritable bowel syndrome, muscle pain, obesity, panic attacks, sinusitis, weight imbalance and other conditions.

Actually, almost everyone has some food allergy and sensitivity, usually as a result of repeated consumption of the same food, general overconsumption or inherited susceptibility. An example of overconsumption in our society is wheat. A morning breakfast cereal with toast, a sandwich for lunch, crackers as a snack, pasta for dinner with cakes and cookies for dessert—this is not at all an uncommon diet routine in our part of the world. Given that many people have a genetic predisposition to wheat sensitivity, developing a sensitivity to wheat gluten is hardly surprising. Celiac disease, a severe condition affecting the digestive system and especially the small intestines, is a genetically inherited overt intolerance of wheat. However, similar symptoms of gas, bloating, polishing of the intestine and malabsorption—all echoing celiac disease—can manifest from gluten sensitivity—the ultimate manifestation of wheat overconsumption. You don't, in other words, need to express the disease genetically or in developed form to be on your way to some equivalent state. Too many food sensitivities can result in your immune system becoming over-reactive, with a resulting abundance of free radicals that can cause body-wide inflammation.

Skin allergy testing determines fixed or immediate responses to food allergies. The doctor may scratch your arm and/or back with suspected allergens and then analyze the welts left behind for their intensity.

But only a blood test can reveal hidden food intolerances. A well-respected and scientifically proven testing protocol called the Enzyme-Linked Immunosorbant Assay provides a useful measurement of antigen (the food in question) and antibody (your immune reaction) concentration, thereby exposing the specific food intolerance. This is an immune reaction governed by a part of the immune system called immunoglobulin gamma (IgG). We're not talking about the difference between good foods, bad foods or even high ORAC foods when we're talking about these immune responses. An IgG reaction can be triggered by broccoli or spinach—hardly bad food choices in other circumstances. The reactions that sensitivities provoke are not as severe as allergies, but nonetheless can cause free radical accumulation, inflammation and a host of other well-known conditions such as those I've mentioned earlier—all induced by oxidative stress. In some cases, refraining from these sensitivity triggers may be enough to lower a person's overall health burden, bringing them under their threshold far enough to remain symptom free.

These tests for food intolerances can look at over 250 different foods, spices and preservatives and their immunological (IgG) relationship. They require only a simple blood test. I've personally seen and dealt with numerous cases of eczema, psoriasis, migraine headaches, fibromyalgia, irritable bowel syndrome and panic attacks that quite literally disappeared once food intolerances were tested for and removed.

Whether a food intolerance results from overconsumption or from an inherited predisposition, remember the first of our four Rs. Dramatic results can sometimes flow from *removing* something from the body rather than putting something into it.

The next stop on the journey to great health is your own antioxidant supplement plan.

CHAPTER 10

YOUR PERSONAL ANTIOXIDANT SUPPLEMENT PLAN

I'm going to devote this entire chapter to the creation of an antioxidant supplement program that you can customize to fit your personal needs.

You may already have embarked on one of the several levels of testing I described in Chapter Five, and if you have, you may be following the supplementation guidelines I offered there. Or perhaps, based on the results of one of these tests (or simply because you've felt it was time for a tune-up), you've started a detoxification program. If so, you've probably completed the first R—*remove*—and you'll soon want to *replenish* and *regenerate*. Or perhaps you want to learn how to supplement on a regular basis to prevent the onset of disease. That's the final R—*repair*.

Whatever your circumstances, if it's supplements you're concerned about, this is the chapter you've been waiting for.

SUPPLEMENTING THE RS
Replenish

The degradation of our gastrointestinal environment is one of the primary points at which our health can be lost. What we now know is that the toxins associated with gastrointestinal dysfunction are frequently absorbed and distributed to other parts of the body. The first thing they do is place a burden on the liver and the immune system. If liver overload occurs, there's going to be spillover, whereby some of the toxins will be passed on to other organs or tissues. This translates into an increasing free radical burden and an increasing need for antioxidants. But once we've detoxified, we need to replenish.

There are three principles we follow if pursuing the regeneration of a detoxified system.

1. We use probiotics and enzymes to encourage better digestion and assimilation of foods.
2. We employ occasional high supplementation doses, followed by regular and established therapeutic doses, of essential fatty acids for improved cell function.
3. We employ single amino acid therapy for the formation of ideal body composition and to increase protection against free radical damage.

The need for regeneration originates from a crucial functional medicine nutrition concept. The frequent malfunction of the digestive and liver detoxification processes, and/or the quality of ingested foods requires that we occasionally aid the body in replenishing certain items at high *therapeutic* amounts in order to ensure optimal function.

As we've discussed, illness can be directly related to problems of the liver detoxification systems and their related influence on immune, nervous and endocrine function and/or nutritional selections in one's diet. Therefore, if we address the health of both the digestive and liver detoxification systems, the body is given the opportunity to reverse almost all degenerative conditions. If the degenerative condition is labelled, for example, chronic fatigue syndrome, diabetes or arthritis, a good homeopathic or naturopathic doctor will first recommend addressing the health of the detoxification and digestive systems (overall gastrointestinal tract). Once the liver detoxification systems are cleared, then the gastrointestinal (GI) tract should be supported and strengthened.

Probiotics

As the name suggests, probiotics are "for life." They are your friendly neighbourhood gut bacteria—the stuff you want in your body. Whereas *anti*biotics kill harmful as well as beneficial bacteria, *pro*biotics in supplement form replenish the beneficial bacteria. Whenever you take antibiotics, have diarrhea or an upset stomach or some type of food poisoning, make sure to take a therapeutic dose of probiotics for anywhere between two weeks to two months, depending on the severity of your symptoms.

Sixty to 80 per cent of our first-line immune defence system is found in our gut, where trillions of *good* bacteria live—good because we need them and good because, for the most part, they cannot cause infection unless they are allowed to escape our gut and enter our bloodstream. These probiotics are cultures of beneficial bacteria that are normally present in a healthy digestive tract. They include *L. acidophilus, B. bifidus, L. planetarium, L. salivarius, L. bulgaricus* and *L. casei.* When these little guys are upset, so too is your immune system.

For over a century, probiotic bacteria—specifically species of the lactobacilli and bifidobacteria genera—have been recognized as potential therapeutic agents. Recently, numerous clinical studies have suggested that these bacterial inhabitants of the human GI tract play an important role in the dietary management of inflammatory bowel diseases (IBD) and chronic degenerative conditions. Such insidious ailments lead inevitably to alarming increases of free radicals in the digestive tract.

Not all probiotics are equal in terms of efficacy. Different probiotic preparations contain different bacterial strains and concentrations. For any probiotic to be effective it must have a high count (in the hundreds of billions of cells) of living bacteria and be able to survive the journey down the GI tract into the colon. The choice of functional strains of micro-organisms is based on criteria established by the scientific community. They must be

- of human origin,
- resistant to stomach acidity and bile salts,
- able to adhere to human intestinal cells,
- able to colonize (even temporarily) the human intestine,
- able to mitigate pathogenic bacteria,
- able to produce antimicrobial substances,
- possessing of immune-balancing ("modulating") properties, and
- proven safe for use by humans.

If you've followed the detoxification program I outline in the section "The Cleanse" in Chapter Seven, I now recommend replenishment by taking about 400 billion probiotic bacteria twice daily following your meals for two weeks. There's debate as to whether they should be broad spectrum (composed of many different strains) or single strains. Some good studies are showing that probiotics survive more effectively and for longer in your gut if you also take "*pre*biotics"—foods that the probiotics thrive on.

Examples are whole grains, onions, bananas, garlic, honey, leeks and artichokes.

Digestive Enzymes

You can't deal with the end-stage problem of free radical burden until you have treated the underlying causes, such as malfunctions in digestion. You are what you eat, but even more important, you become what you absorb.

Enzymes are manufactured in our digestive tracts from the moment we think about or smell food. Hydrochloric acid is made in our stomach and digests protein; pancreatic enzymes are manufactured in our pancreas and digest starches, sugars and certain proteins; bile is produced in the liver and held in the gall bladder and is responsible for breaking down fats.

When we eat a heavy restaurant meal or our mother's famous meat loaf and afterwards it feels like a brick in our stomach, odds are we aren't producing enough enzymes to break down that food. That's when supplemental enzymes can help. But when we employ enzymes in capsule form as supplements, their effects can and should last weeks to months, depending on the health challenges they must confront.

Enzymes also have a broad variety of specific therapeutic applications as anti-inflammatory, anticoagulant and antithrombolytic agents, and as replacements for metabolic deficiencies. Here are a few:

Proteolytic enzymes have been widely used as anti-inflammatory and antiedema agents. In clinical practice, I use a brand called Wobenzym-N, and patients report wonderful results, with many of their digestive challenges resolved and even arthritis pain gone.

Papain enzyme derives from the pineapple. In capsular form, it has been shown to produce marked reduction of obstetrical inflammation and swelling and of the edema following dental surgery.

Deoxyribonuclease, an enzyme that degrades nucleic acid, has recently been investigated as a mucous-thinning agent for use in patients with chronic bronchitis. Although effective in producing liquefaction of secretions, it offers no advantage over more commonly recommended agents such as the antioxidant *N*-acetyl-L-cysteine.

The enzyme *lysozyme* breaks down bacterial cell walls. Accordingly, it has been used as an antibacterial agent, usually in combination with standard antibiotics.

The proteolytic enzymes *trypsin* and *chymotrypsin* (both of which are in Wobenzym-N) have been successfully used in the treatment of postoperative trauma, athletic injuries and sciatica.

Hyaluronidase exerts action by allowing diffusion of vital molecules through the barrier of normally impermeable connective tissue in joint tissue.

A good broad-spectrum digestive enzyme is one that provides 1,000,000 USP units or more of protease activity, 5,000 USP units or more of amylase activity and 1,000 USP units or more of lipase activity. Even if you haven't tried the cleanse, take two capsules with every meal for two months and see if you experience better digestion and improved energy.

Essential Fatty Acids

We've already spoken a lot about some of the benefits of omega-3 fatty acids, but these essential fats have another short-term but crucial role to play.

Toxins can affect any part of us. However, their toxic influence may be greatest on our brains and nervous systems. After a detoxification program, I recommend you increase your daily dose of fish oils for a few weeks. Fish oils at this dose are what I refer to as gut rehab and brain juice. Taking therapeutic doses for two weeks will not only have a rehabilitative effect on your liver and blood, but will also help improve the quality of stool and generally "Draino" the pipes.

Take 10 mL three times daily of the cleanest brand—Ascenta's NutraSea oil, for example—for 2 weeks, then reduce to 5 mL twice daily with food. Avoid this therapeutic level dose if you are on blood-thinning medication. Cut back slowly if you experience diarrhea.

Single Amino Acid Therapy

This can be an extremely important part of replenishment. The lining of your gut is where your body selects foods for absorption and certain amino acids have a natural ability to repair the gut lining. These are glutamine, arginine and cysteine in the form of N-acetylcysteine (NAC). Glutamine has the ability to "astringe" the mucous membrane of the intestine and restore it to its proper selective-absorption state. NAC together with L-arginine and C-glutamine alleviate many cases of inflammatory bowel syndrome by promoting the healing of colon inflammation and resolving a condition know as "leaky gut syndrome" (which has been gaining recent attention for causing those food intolerances I wrote about in the previous chapter.)

Administration of these three amino acids range in dose

depending on the situation. After detoxification, take glutamine at 5,000 to 10,000 mg per day, arginine at 1,000 to 2,000 mg per day in a slow-release form and NAC at 500 to 1,000 mg per day, all on an empty stomach.

Regenerate

Following the removal of toxins and the replenishment of crucial probiotics, we embark upon the third R, *regeneration*, that is, short-term antioxidant support—therapeutic intervention that targets the body's cells. Because individual requirements have a strong bearing on this sort of therapy, you should test your urine in order to determine the dosages that are ideal for you at this stage. The home-based antioxidant urine test we looked at in Chapter Five (part of the Bryce Wylde's Antioxidant Test Kit) measures the damaged cell material in your body that arises as a result of free radical activity *during* the detoxification process and after.

This test accurately measures how effectively antioxidants in your diet and inherent in your body have neutralized free radicals during your detox routine. The antioxidant urine test returns results scored from Levels 1 to 5. Level 1 is the lowest, and is a great result to see. Level 2 is low, and means you're doing well but could do even better. Levels 3 to 5 are medium, high and very high: you've got some work to do in neutralizing the free radical attack that is currently under way in your body, and you need fairly heavy antioxidant support. With these results in hand, see my recommendations in "Step II: The Antioxidant Prescription" where I correlate urine test levels with your score on "Step 1: The Free Radical Calculation," and you'll be well on your way to determining whether or not to increase your antioxidant intake over the short term to support your body's cellular regeneration.

Regeneration is not the last step. We now move on to the final R, *repair*—the basis of a lifetime regimen.

Repair

As we saw in Chapter Six, our bodies are in a continuous process of damage and repair. Even when we've completed a therapeutic regeneration cycle, we constantly need cellular repair and maintenance. We now know a great deal about the power of antioxidants to accomplish this ongoing repair, and in the sections that follow I'm going to describe a supplementation program you'll want to follow whether you decide to do the detoxification or not. The essential question is this: How much supplementation?

A Customized Antioxidant Supplement Program

Practitioners of natural medicine increasingly understand that antioxidant nutrients do more than prevent classical deficiency diseases and help the young to grow and the old to maintain their health. They protect against most diseases associated with aging. As we have seen, at optimal levels, they may protect against nearly *all* disease.

The idea that you can enjoy better health through the use of antioxidant supplements is difficult for many to accept. It seems that nature should provide for all of our needs. The operative word here is "needs." For what? Procreation? Average health? Maximum lifespan free of disease? Because few of us are afflicted with what I affectionately call the "George Burns syndrome"— abuse your organs and live to a hundred—our more average genes need antioxidant nutrients in high amounts to protect us against cellular and genetic damage that leads to disease and shortened lives.

Since recommended daily intake (RDI) levels for various nutrients are obtained by extrapolating data from short-term laboratory animal experiments based on normal growth rates, and since RDI is intended to suggest the needs for "average" health for the "average" person, RDIs have little relevance to optimal daily allowance (ODA) for health and longevity. Anyway, few of us manage even the recommended daily intake levels, and even if we do make a tremendous effort to eat a fruit- and veggie-filled diet, these foods no longer contain the antioxidants they once did.

ODAs attempt to take into account our nutritional needs for the optimization of our immune systems, the prevention of cancer and heart disease, and a whole lot more. Put it this way, when it comes to vitamin C, we're not looking to avoid scurvy with 60 mg/day (the RDI of vitamin C); we're looking to optimize our immune systems with thousands of milligrams per day (the ODA of vitamin C). Let me go further. If we consume less than optimal ranges (ODA) of the antioxidant nutrients, we run the risk of heart disease, cancer, arthritis and anything else our genetic predispositions can dish out. Respected studies have shown that even if we eat well and take a simple multivitamin/mineral supplement, our risk of disease is not so very different from those who take no multivitamins whatsoever!

In our supplement program, we'll employ *therapeutic*-range supplementation to achieve optimal health. In the course of doing this, we're going to perform a further antioxidant assessment by calculating your approximate exposure to free radicals. You'll then be able to write out your own antioxidant prescription.

The Antioxidant Assessment

Below, you'll find the assessment, which is in two parts. Photocopy "Step I: The Free Radical Calculation," and fill it in. It's simple. Each row represents a health variable. For each variable there are three possible levels, to which we've assigned either 1 point, 2 points or 3 points. Add up the points in each row to get your score for that health variable. For example, if you're 45, if your BMI is 33 and if the average age of your deceased grandparents is 74, your score for those three variables is 8 points. If you're simply unsure which level fits you best for a given variable, score a minimum of 2 points for that given box. Two variables, BMI and Stress, require a little additional calculation that I explain beneath the template. When you're done, total the points in the right-hand column to get your total score. The score is not purely scientific, but it does represent a crude description of your likely free radical levels and is based on years of observation and practice.

Testing yourself, either with a professional in the field of natural medicine or with an at-home urine kit such as my own, will always give you more accurate results than this simple assessment exercise. But by combining the two—this assessment *and* the urine test—with a dash of common sense, you'll have new insight into *why* free radicals are accumulating in you.

THE ANTIOXIDANT ASSESSMENT

STEP I: THE FREE RADICAL CALCULATION

Variable	1 point	2 points	3 points	Score for this row
1. Age	Below 30	31–50	51+	_____
2. *BMI	19–24.9 (healthy)	25–29.9 (overweight)	30+ (obese)	_____
3. Average age of deceased grandparents	80 or more	75–80	Less than 75	_____

*Calculate your approximate BMI. (A body impedance analysis done by machine is more accurate, but we'll use BMI for the purpose of this exercise.) Record your height in meters and multiply that number by itself. Then weigh yourself in kilograms. Then divide the weight by the number obtained in the first multiplication step. For example, you might be 1.6 m (5 ft., 3 in.) tall and weigh 65 kg (143 lb.). The calculation would then be:
1.6 x 1.6 = 2.56. Your BMI would be 65 divided by 2.56 = 25.39.
NOTE: If your BMI is 35+ and you have a waist size of over 100 cm (40 in.) (men) and 90 cm (35 in.) (women), you are considered to be at especially high risk of many and varied health problems. If your BMI is 40+, you are considered to be seriously obese and at a very serious risk of health problems.

Variable	1 point	2 points	3 points	Score for this row
4. Immediate family history (parents and siblings)	Unremarkable generally healthy	Obesity, asthma eczema, digestive issues, allergies	Diabetes, heart disease, cancer major psycho-logical disorder, autoimmune disease	_____
5. Face and body skin appearance	Very few wrinkles	Moderate amount of wrinkles and moles/freckles	Heavily wrinkled, high degree of moles	_____
6. Body type	Fit (hourglass shape to well proportioned)	Pear-shaped (thin upper body and large hips buttocks and thighs)	Apple-shaped (excessive abdo-minal weight)	_____
7. Exercise	3–6	7–15	Less than 2 hours, score as above. 16-30 hours: if you exercise this much score 5 points in this category.	_____
8. Residence pollution levels	Mountains, rural clean	Suburban (uptown)	Urban (downtown)	_____
9. Workplace pollution levels	Clean, filtered air; frequent inspections	Moderate (i.e., I sit in earshot of a photocopier and there are no windows.)	High (I am working in direct contact with tox-ins such as paints or petrochemicals or other chemicals or I am a profes-sional working with toxins, e.g., a dentist.)	_____
10. Air travel	Fewer than 6 flights/year	6–24 flights /year	24+ flights /year	_____
11. Age of Dwelling	2–10 years	10–25 + years	More than 25 or less than 2 years	
12. Stress levels (To determine, use the questionnaire below)	5–10	10–15	15–20	_____

Variable	1 point	2 points	3 points	Score for this row
13. Daily use of cosmetic and aesthetic products	Minimal (i.e., use non-perfumed soap, deodorant and body lotion)	Moderate (i.e., as for Minimal plus perfume or cologne and hair gel/spray)	Excessive (i.e., as for Moderate plus facial makeup and nail polish)	_____
14. Cell phone use	Less than 1 hour/day	Between 1–3 hours/day	More than 3 hours/day	_____
15. Over-the-counter use of medications	Minimal (only in emergency)	Moderate (every time I get sick)	Frequent (At the slightest sniffle or headache I down a Tylenol.)	_____
16. Prescription drug use	None	Moderate (1–3 prescriptions)	High (3 or more prescriptions)	_____
17. History of sun exposure or use of tanning	Minimal (monthly, i.e., only on holidays; otherwise skin is original colour)	Moderate (weekly, (weekly, i.e., will sunbathe when I get a chance)	High (2 or more times/week, beds i.e., I sunbathe and /or use tanning beds frequently.)	_____
18. Tobacco use	Not at all	Social (1 or 2 cigarettes on rare occasions, or a cigar)	I am a smoker or I am exposed second-hand smoke.	_____

TOTAL SCORE _____   _____

SCORE YOUR STRESS LEVELS.
For an evaluation of physical and emotional stress, count the number of times you answer yes to the following questions, and then score accordingly in the calculator above.

Yes/No

1. Do you have trouble getting along with your co-workers?   _____
2. Do you hide from others how you are feeling?   _____
3. Do you suffer from constipation or diarrhea?   _____
4. Do you get jealous of others?   _____
5. Do you get colds/flu frequently?   _____

6. When you fall ill, does it often take more than four days to recover? _____
7. Do you frequently crave sweet things to eat? _____
8. Do you suffer from frequent headaches? _____
9. Are you quick to anger? _____
10. Do you feel that you are frequently under a major deadline? _____
11. Do you feel sluggish at the beginning of the day? _____
12. Do you often feel lonely? _____
13. Do you drink more than one drink/day (females) or two drinks/day (males)? _____
14. Does your heart often pound or flutter? _____
15. Do you have difficulty sleeping? _____
16. When conflict arises do you over-react or do you generally have a bad temper? _____
17. Do you have difficulty concentrating? _____
18. Do you have allergy flare-ups or frequent hives on your skin? _____
19. Do you sweat excessively? _____
20. Are you most often in a bad mood? _____

Total times you answered yes to any of the above: _____

Now for the easy part. The Free Radical Calculation generates a minimum possible score of 18 and a maximum possible score of 56. Take your total score from the calculation and apply it to "Part II: The Antioxidant Prescription" on pages 179 to determine the supplement levels that will comprise your personalized antioxidant supplement program. The lowest recommended intake for the various antioxidants represents slightly more than the amount of antioxidant obtained from an optimal diet in combination with a quality multivitamin. Current research suggests that protection from free radical exposure requires higher levels of antioxidants than are necessary for simple deficiency protection. Without the benefit of specific testing, this assessment tool can suggest only the approximate range for your personal therapeutic dose of antioxidants. If your score is between 25 and 34, for example, the calculator suggests your vitamin E levels should be 800 IU daily. You may decide to use a good multivitamin/mineral as a base to your program, but if your multi contains only 200 IU, you'll want to add another 600 IU to your daily regimen.

The best way to take these antioxidants is with food, twice daily, morning and evening. Remember to take as many of these antioxidants together as possible—synergy is the key. A few days without them won't do much harm, so if you run out of some, wait until you can restock before you resume the program. In the meanwhile, continue your daily multi.

Again, this is a rule-of-thumb calculator. You can more precisely determine your antioxidant supplement needs, regardless of age or lifestyle, by accessing a medical testing facility in consultation with your health-care provider. Together, you can order up any or all of the testing we discussed in Chapter Five. With those more accurate test results in hand, you can better track how the following prescriptive action plan for nutrition and supplementation works and continues to work for you over time by retesting to assess any necessary changes. Depending on the laboratory retests, and taking everything known about your health into account, you could decide how to use the antioxidants I list in the antioxidant prescription chart below. Or you can use my home test, and use the recommendations I've made on the chart below, checking in with your holistic health-care practitioner.

DO NOT take any antioxidant supplements if you are unsure of how they may interact with any medication you may be taking. It is always best to seek the advice of a qualified physician.

STEP II: THE ANTIOXIDANT PRESCRIPTION

YOUR TOTAL SCORE FROM THE FREE RADICAL ASSESSMENT (Bryce Wylde's Antioxidant Test Kit levels)	18–24 (Level 1 Clear)	25–34 (Level 2 Light Pink)	35–44 (Level 3 Magenta)	45+ (Levels 4–5 Red–Dark Red)
			UNITS DAILY	
*Vitamin E (IU) (D-alpha-tocopherol succinate)	400	800	1,200	1,600
*Vitamin C (mg)	250	500	1,000	2,000
*Beta-carotene (IU)	10,000	20,000	35,000	50,000
Vitamin D	1,000	2,000	3,000	4,000
Coenzyme Q_{10} (mg)	30	60	120	180
Acetyl-L-carnitine (mg)	500	1,000	1,500	2,000
N-acetylcysteine (g)	100	200	300	400
*Selenium (mcg) (L-selenomethionne)	200	300	450	600
Zinc (mg) (citrate)	15	25	35	50
Manganese (mg) (gluconate)	5	10	20	30
Alpha-lipoic 100 acid (mg)	200	300	400	600
Lycopene (mg)	20	40	60	100
IP-6 (mg)	100	200	300	400
Procyanidins (mg) (i.e., pycnogenol at 75% proanthocyanidins by weight)	50	100	150	200
Catechins (mg) (i.e., green tea extract)	250	500	1,000	1,500
Melatonin (mg) (taken 1 hour before bed for no longer than 3 months at a time with a break of 1 month in between)	1	2	3	6

*These are the antioxidant ACES.

Inside Our Supplements

I hope you'll want to know more about these substances I'm suggesting you take. They are safe and proven, but this critical attitude will stand you in good stead as you enter the brave new world of therapeutic supplementation. Before we end this chapter, I want to offer you a brief summary of what each supplement/antioxidant can do for you beyond simply neutralizing free radicals.

The following information is based in part on the work done by Jeff M. Jellin of the Natural Medicines Comprehensive Database (NMCD). This database, which relies mostly on U.S. research, offers a wealth of qualified information on natural medicines, including sections on safety, efficacy, mechanism of action, and drug and food interactions for each listed substance and, in many cases, brands. I've used this source of information because it is the most trusted available, and I believe that despite some variations in disease prevalence in Canada, the UK and other Western nations, the findings are equally applicable.

VITAMIN E

A broad class of related natural chemicals called tocopherols comprise the fat-soluble antioxidants we call vitamin E. Alpha-tocopherol is generally regarded as the most active form of vitamin E in humans, though new research is showing the importance of other forms of the vitamin. By definition, the proper levels of all vitamins are essential to human health, but good evidence now links vitamin E intake to the prevention of eye diseases, including cataracts, glaucoma and macular degeneration; other studies may link the vitamin to the prevention or delay of both Alzheimer's and Parkinson's diseases. Meanwhile, ongoing research is exploring vitamin E's role in the prevention of heart disease, cancer and a host of other diseases. You may have noticed some studies in the last few years that downplay the effect of vitamin E. I implore that you pay little attention to them. These studies were indeed carried out by recognized groups but were incomplete and in my opinion irresponsible. They appeared to suggest that vitamin E at higher doses—doses I regard as therapeutic—could cause more harm then good. But these were "all-cause mortality" studies, which means that if you were one of the subjects taking vitamin E and got hit by a bus, the researchers would have counted you as having died from taking vitamin E. Getting hit by a bus or dying from natural causes is nothing whatsoever to do with vitamin E. Most scientific evidence suggests vitamin E is an excellent antioxidant, and when you need more of it, it's crucial to obtain it through a supplement.

If you decide to have a vaccination, and are 16 or older, take 8,000 IU of vitamin E daily for at least a week before your shot. Also make sure that you get enough sleep that same week, at least eight hours a night. Both tactics have been shown to enhance the effects of immunization.

Vitamin E Precautions: Consult a specialist before using vitamin E if you have

- *just undergone a procedure called angioplasty,*
- *been told you have low levels of vitamin K,*
- *an eye condition called retinitis pigmentosa,*
- *a blood clotting disorder, and/or*
- *head and neck cancer.*

Possible Vitamin E Interactions with Prescription Medications
Consult a specialist before using vitamin E if you are taking

- *cyclosporine (Neoral, Sandimmune),*
- *warfarin (Coumadin),*
- *medications changed by the liver (cytochrome P-450 3A4 [CYP3A4] substrates),*
- *certain medications for cancer (chemotherapy),*

- *certain medications used for lowering cholesterol (statins), and/or*
- *certain medications that slow blood clotting (anticoagu-lant/antiplatelet drugs).*

VITAMIN C

The fame of the powerful antioxidant vitamin C stems partly from the fact that it is an essential nutrient in almost all living creatures, and almost all living creatures produce it—humans being an exception. Without dietary vitamin C, humans develop a terrible disease called scurvy, but many researchers believe that the doses needed to prevent scurvy are insufficient for maintaining good health. Good studies have linked the vitamin to such diverse health benefits as preventing lead absorption, preventing organ failure in surgery patients, reducing the devastating effects of strokes and improving the quality of health in patients. In this book, we've concerned ourselves with the potent antioxidant effects of this vitamin, and it's safe to say, the more research that is carried out, the more valuable vitamin C is recognized to be.

What has changed recently for a number of clinicians is the notion of megadosing. New studies suggest that *therapeutic* effects of vitamin C may be achieved from as low a dosage as 250 mg/day. I personally think that at least 1,000 mg/day—and sometimes more—is necessary for most people to maintain ideal levels.

Controlled studies comparing schizophrenics with people without the disorder have shown that schizoprenics had lower vitamin C levels in their blood. They were also found to need much higher amounts of vitamin C than the average person.

Vitamin C Precautions: Consult a specialist before using vitamin C if you have

- *a blood-iron disorder, including conditions called thalassemia and hemochromatosis;*
- *kidney stones or a history of kidney stones;*
- *a metabolic deficiency called "glucose-6-phosphate dehydrogenase deficiency" (G6PDD); or*
- *a blood disorder called sickle cell disease.*

Possible Vitamin C Interactions with Prescription Medications: Consult a specialist before taking vitamin C if you are taking the following:

- Warfarin (Coumadin): *Warfarin is used to slow blood clotting. Large amounts of vitamin C might decrease the effectiveness of warfarin. Decreasing the effectiveness of warfarin might increase the risk of clotting. If you're on warfarin, be sure to have your blood checked regularly. The dose may need to be changed.*

BETA-CAROTENE

Renowned for the yellow colour it imparts to carrots and for which it's named, beta-carotene is a so-called carotene pigment found in many colourful vegetables and converted by the body to the essential vitamin A. Deficiencies of vitamin A cause deleterious changes to vision and the skin, and the vitamin has been used in trials to reduce photosensitivities, cataracts, age-related macular degeneration and a host of other conditions.

Studies have shown that if you smoke you shouldn't supplement with beta-carotene as it may increase your chances of developing lung cancer. For non-smokers, beta-carotene is beneficial for the skin, reducing oil and keratin production.

Beta-Carotene Precautions: Consult a specialist before using beta-carotene if you

- *are pregnant or breastfeeding;*
- *smoke;*
- *have been exposed to high levels of asbestos; and/or*
- *are going to have angioplasty, a heart procedure.*

Possible Beta-Carotene Interactions with Prescription Medications: Consult a specialist before using beta-carotene if you are taking

- *medications used for lowering cholesterol (statins).*

COENZYME Q_{10} (CoQ_{10})

We encountered this coenzyme in Chapter Two as one of the powerful antioxidants that defend our cells against free radical activity. In another form, CoQ_{10} plays a critical metabolic role as part of the process by which our cells' mitochondria convert nutrients into 95 per cent of the energy we need. Although the bodies of younger people are able to manufacture CoQ_{10}, older people may not, making it essential to health. As a supplement, CoQ_{10} has recently shown great promise in the treatment or prevention of migraine headaches, heart diesease, cancer, neurodegenerative diseases and many other conditions.

CoQ_{10} is an important antioxidant in the prevention of heart disease and ameliorates the side effects of heart medication. Some studies have shown that it also slows the progression of early-stage Parkinson's disease.

CoQ_{10} Precautions: Consult a specialist before using CoQ_{10} if

- *you are pregnant or breastfeeding.*

Possible CoQ_{10} Interactions with Prescription Medications: Consult a specialist before using CoQ_{10} if you are taking

- *certain medications for cancer (chemotherapy),*
- *medications for high blood pressure (antihypertensive drugs), and/or*
- *warfarin (Coumadin).*

ACETYL-L-CARNITINE
This is an antioxidant that can increase energy and aid in weight loss.

Acetyl-L-Carnitine
Acetyl-l-carnitine is a dual-acting antioxidant and amino acid, known for protecting nerve cells. It also enhances brain communication by sweeping up the free radical mess inside your brain.

Acetyl-L-Carnitine Precautions: Consult a specialist before using acetyl-L-carnitine if you

- *are pregnant or breastfeeding,*
- *have had seizures, and/or*
- *have thyroid problems.*

Possible Acetyl-L-Carnitine Interactions with Prescription Medications: Consult a specialist before using acetyl-L-carnitine if you are taking either of the following:

- Acenocoumarol (Sintrom). *This is an important warning because acenocoumarol is used to slow blood clotting. Acetyl-L-carnitine may increase the effectiveness of aceno-coumarol. Increasing the effectiveness of acenocoumarol may slow blood clotting too much. The dose of your acenocoumarol may need to be changed.*
- *Warfarin (Coumadin).*

N-ACETYLCYSTEINE (NAC)

NAC is a form of the amino acid cysteine, although unlike ordinary cysteine, which occurs only in protein foods, *N*-acetylcysteine is produced in the human body. It plays an important role in the liver's natural detoxifying activities and is metabolized as glutathione, a potent antioxidant, chemical detoxifier and immune system component that cannot itself be easily absorbed orally. For this reason, NAC is now under serious investigation as a supplement. In hospital settings, NAC is important in treating patients with acetaminophen (e.g., Tylenol) poisoning and is one of the most effective available chelating agents, those valuable chemicals that can clear the body of heavy metals. NAC also acts to break up mucus, and so has proved useful in the treatment of such diseases as influenza and bronchitis. Its usefulness in cancer and many other diseases is currently under investigation.

Taking *N*-acetylcysteine thins mucous secretions, which helps inflamed and stuffy sinuses and lungs drain more effectively.

N-Acetylcysteine Precautions: Consult a specialist before using N-acetylcysteine if you

- *are pregnant or breastfeeding,*
- *are allergic to acetylcysteine, and/or*
- *have asthma.*

Possible N-acetylcysteine Interactions with Prescription Medications: Consult a specialist before using N-acetylcysteine if you are taking the following:

- Nitroglycerin. *This is an important caution because nitroglycerin can dilate blood vessels and increase blood flow. Taking N-acetylcysteine seems to increase the effects of nitroglycerin. This may cause increased chance of side effects, including headache, dizziness and light-headedness.*

SELENIUM

Selenium is trace metallic element found in soil, water and some foods and is essential to human metabolism in small amounts. As a supplement, it is being actively investigated for the prevention of prostate cancer and possibly some other cancers, since many cancer sufferers have been shown to have low selenium levels. Selenium has also been the subject of study for the prevention and treatment of many diseases, and some early results are encouraging.

Selenium is not a true antioxidant but rather a trace mineral. But it recycles antioxidants and reduces inflammation in conditions such as acne.

Selenium Precautions: Consult a specialist before using selenium if you

- *are a man with fertility problems. Selenium might decrease the ability of sperm to move, which could reduce fertility, and/or*
- *have or have had skin cancer.*

Possible Selenium Interactions with Prescription Medications: Consult a specialist before using selenium if you are taking

- *sedative medications (barbiturates).*

ZINC

The metallic element zinc is an essential nutrient, not only for humans but also for most forms of life. Its role in uncounted biological processes and in the biological signalling between cells is under intense and growing investigation. Only truly varied diets are likely to contain enough zinc, a worrying fact when we consider that zinc deficiency leads to a wide variety of conditions from acne to stunted brain development and has been implicated in everything from anorexia nervosa to night blindness. The consequences are especially serious for children of zinc-deficient mothers. Like selenium, zinc is often used in conjunction with antioxidants, and a list of traditional and recently confirmed applications would be far too long to consider here. Think antidandruff shampoo. Think cold-and-flu remedy. And on and on.

Note: Like zinc, the metal copper is an indispensable nutrient in trace amounts, though it is toxic in larger amounts. We normally get enough of this through vegetable sources and, unfortunately, tap water due to copper piping. Because copper and zinc may compete for uptake in the digestive system, an excess of one may mean a deficiency of the other. Copper is used to treat anemia due to copper deficiency, and zinc-induced copper deficiency. Some supplement specialists use copper to improve wound healing, osteoarthritis and osteoporosis.

Zinc has antiviral effects and zinc lozenges or nasal spray may be very effective for colds and flu.

Zinc Precautions: Consult a specialist before using zinc if you have

- *HIV (human immunodeficiency virus).*

Possible Zinc Interactions with Prescription Medications: Consult a specialist before using zinc if you are taking

- *quinolone or tetracycline antibiotics,*
- *cisplatin (Platinol-AQ), and/or*
- *penicillamine.*

MANGANESE

Like selenium, zinc and copper, the metal manganese is a critical nutrient, though toxic in excess. Manganese is intimately involved in the antioxidation process within our cells' mitochrondria. It plays an important role in bone and cartilage development and in wound healing. For all these reasons and others, manganese is a widely recommended supplement. Like copper and zinc, manganese and iron may compete for absorption, so that excess iron may inhibit the body's uptake of manganese.

Like selenium, manganese is a trace mineral, not an antioxidant, but it is necessary for the function of enzyme systems involved with energy production, blood sugar control, fatty acid synthesis, thyroid hormone function, connective tissue and bone formation, and the healing of sprains and strains. Again like selenium, it helps antioxidants recycle themselves.

Manganese Precautions: Consult a specialist before using manganese if you

• *have liver problems.*

Possible Manganese Interactions with Prescription Medications
Consult a specialist before using manganese if you are taking

• *quinolone or tetracycline antibiotics.*

ALPHA-LIPOIC ACID (ALA)

ALA is an essential nutrient, a cofactor in many enzymatic actions and a potent antioxidant. Its promise as a supplement was first revealed in a successful 1970s study to treat acute and severe liver damage. Since the 1990s, in conjunction with antioxidants, it has shown promise in combatting certain metastatic cancers. More recently, in combination with L-carnitine, it has been shown to improve memory performance and to delay structural mitochondrial decay.

Alpha-lipoic acid is an antioxidant that can take on the role of vitamin C. It also improves insulin sensitivity, which means it can help control blood sugar levels. It reduces the symptoms of diabetic neuropathy too.

Alpha-Lipoic Acid Precautions: Consult a specialist before using alpha-lipoic acid if you

- *are pregnant or breastfeeding,*
- *use alcohol excessively,*
- *have thiamine deficiency, and/or*
- *have thyroid disease.*

Possible Alpha Lipoic Acid Interactions with Prescription Medications: Consult a specialist before using alpha-lipoic acid if you are taking

- *certain medications for cancer (chemotherapy).*

LYCOPENE

Like beta-carotene, lycopene is a carotene, an important phytochemical (a chemical derived from plants) whose molecule contains no oxygen and is therefore a potent oxygen absorber, that is, an antioxidant. Lycopene is currently subject to intensive trials to confirm its cardiovascular effects and its usefulness in preventing cancer, especially prostate cancer.

Lycopene is an antioxidant that comes from tomatoes and is useful in the prevention of many forms of cancer, including prostate cancer. A research study also found that more than half the people with exercise-induced asthma in the trial had significantly fewer asthma symptoms after taking lycopene daily for a week, compared to those who took the placebo.

Lycopene Precautions: Consult a specialist before using lycopene if you

- *are pregnant or breastfeeding or*
- *have active prostate cancer.*

Possible Lycopene Interactions with Prescription Medications

- *No known interactions.*

INOSITOL HEXAPHOSPHATE or PHYTIC ACID (IP-6)
Many plants use phytic acid to store phosphorus, and it is found in the hulls of nuts, seeds and grains, from which it is freed by cooking. The IP-6 form is a powerful chelating agent that is useful for removing metals from the body, but it may also remove essential nutrient metals when these are deficient in the diet, as is often the case with small children. Phytic acid's antioxidant and chelating properties may make it one of nature's most effective agents against colon cancer and possibly other cancers.

Research shows that inositol hexaphosphate reduces common kidney stone formation, where crystals are formed of calcium-oxalate.

Inositol Hexaphosphate Precautions: Consult a specialist before using inositol hexaphosphate if you

- *are pregnant or breastfeeding,*
- *have a low iron condition called iron-deficiency anemia, and/or*
- *have a bone condition called osteoporosis or osteopenia.*

Possible Inositol Hexaphosphate Interactions with Prescription Medications: Consult a specialist before using inositol hexaphosphate if you are taking

- *medications that slow blood clotting (anticoagulant/antiplatelet drugs).*

PROCYANIDINS

Procyanidins are condensed tannins, the agents responsible for the familiar puckering taste of much young red wine. This group of phytochemicals has received a lot of publicity because it is believed to be partly responsible for the benefits of the Mediterranean diet. Most researchers now agree that procyanidins are linked to a reduced risk of coronary heart disease and to generally lower mortality. Grape procyanidins were first classed as a vitamin (vitamin P) when discovered in the 1930s, and a recent study suggests that procyanidins' antioxidant capabilities are twenty times higher than vitamin C and fifty times higher than vitamin E. The seeds and skins of red grapes are among the most abundant sources of procyanidins. As a result red grape juice (and wine) are rich in these agents, though they are not found in high concentrations in grape seed oil.

An antioxidant made of procyanidins obtained from the bark of Pinus maritime, the European coastal pine, has been shown in multiple studies to be effective in the treatment of varicose veins.

Procyanidins Precautions:

- *None known.*

Possible Procyanidins Interactions with Prescription Medications:

- *None known.*

CATECHINS

Catechins belong to a group of phytochemicals called flavonoids and are found in numerous foods, including cacao, wine, vegetables and fruits. They're most abundant, however, in the tea plant, *Camellia sinensis,* and thus in most teas. A wide range of health benefits have been linked to catechins. For example, they reduce the risk of stroke, heart failure, cancer and diabetes—four of the deadliest diseases in the developed world. It has been argued that the catechins should be officially listed as a vitamin group.

In studies catechins have been shown to be helpful in treating acute and chronic hepatitis.

Catechins Precautions:

- *None known.*

Possible Catechins Interactions with Prescription Medications:

- *None known.*

MELATONIN

Metatonin is a hormone found in virtually all living creatures. Its primary role is to regulate the daily cycles of various biological functions; in humans its release is triggered by darkness, which causes the pineal gland to release it. It is also a powerful antioxidant. As a supplement, the enzyme is used for jet lag, insomnia, shift-work disorder, circadian rhythm disorders in the blind and benzodiazepine and nicotine withdrawal. Melatonin is also being tested for its effectiveness in treating Alzheimer's disease, tinnitus, depression, chronic fatigue syndrome, fibromyalgia, headaches and irritable bowel syndrome. It is presently also under investigation for potential in preventing certain cancers.

Melatonin is a hormone produced by your brain that is responsible for regulating your bio-rhythms or internal clock. It's one of the most powerful antioxidants, and it helps slow down the aging process. It also prevents breast and prostate cancers, relieves cluster headaches, and ameliorates radiation exposure and seasonal affective disorder.

Melatonin Precautions: Consult a specialist before using melatonin if you

- *are pregnant or breastfeeding,*
- *have high blood pressure,*
- *have had a seizure,*
- *have diabetes,*
- *have certain forms of cancer, and/or*
- *have certain forms of depression.*

Possible Melatonin Interactions with Prescription Medications: Consult a specialist before using melatonin if you are taking

- *certain sedative medications (CNS depressants),*
- *nifedipine GITS (Procardia XL),*
- *medications that decrease the immune system (immunosuppressants), and/or*
- *fluvoxamine (Luvox).*

Last Word on Supplements

Medical technology—from brain surgery to quadruple bypasses—has brought life and hope to desperately sick people. For example, the cleansing power of dialysis machines has given patients whose kidneys have failed extra years of life. Myriad examples illustrate medical technology's power to extend the average human lifespan in the face of a vast range of traumas and diseases.

But now imagine this: These people—long before they fall ill—take a number of simple gelatin-coated capsules that contain powerful and carefully tailored food-derived nutrients and they also eat foods rich in antioxidants. They do this every day of their lives. As a result, they don't develop the diseases that medical technology is designed to rescue them from! Imagine such a scenario and then consider that it's no longer science fiction. With the knowledge we now possess, health insurance—at least in part—is increasingly available in a bottle. The rest is up to us.

CHAPTER 11

YOUR PERSONAL ANTIOXIDANT EXERCISE PLAN

If it were that simple, I'd say "not to worry, just exercise regularly any old how and you'll be fine." But studies are finding that many long-distance runners and weight lifters end up with early hip and knee replacements and arthritis. The latest science suggests that we need to move it much more often than we do, but we also need to stop injuring our joints by *over*exercising or exercising improperly.

Think about boxers. They're supposedly superhealthy and strong—and actually *are* for a few years—flaunting 10 per cent body fat and abdominal muscles you could scrub your laundry on. But when they retire they can end up brain-damaged as the result of a stroke or otherwise disabled and confined to a wheelchair while the hired help wipes away their involuntary slobber. When it comes to free radical damage, other forms of impact exercise—like running marathons and bench pressing twice your body weight—can be almost as damaging to the system as getting slammed in the cranium at a hundred miles in a boxing ring. For many of us, alternating between sedentary life and (for those who *are* making an effort) weekend-warrior exercise routines can also result in injury. We sit in front of the computer all week, and then come the weekend, we attempt to run marathons or go camping carrying 35 kg (80 lb.) bags, trusting that we are making up for lost exercise. Strenuous exercise can cause a chemical called xanthine oxidase to build up in our muscles and joints. The creation of free radicals from the damage by xanthine oxidase is extremely detrimental to our overall health.

You may have heard of gout. Xanthine oxidase, it just so happens, is largely responsible for this debilitating and painful (though usually temporary) condition.

Some interesting studies, comparing marathon runners who did and did not take antioxidant supplements, were reported by the journal *Proceedings* of the Fisher Institute for Medical Research in August 2003 (vol. 3, no.1). Antioxidant protection appeared to be powerfully enhanced by the use of free radical-fighting "glyconutritional" supplementation. The bodies of supplemented runners appeared to be protected for several days after the marathon run. However, for those subjects not receiving the glyconutritional sports nutrition, the damaging effects of free radicals appeared to remain in the body for about five days. These control subjects consistently excreted higher concentrations of free radical by-products as compared with those receiving the glyconutritional supplement.

Not exercising at all contributes far more to the body's free radical load and is far worse for our overall health.

Heart disease—along with artery lining dysfunction and plaque formation—is a proven consequence of inactivity. Our predominantly sedentary lifestyle—not to mention over-consumption—prompts our doctors to warn us so frequently to either *start* exercising (or keep up the good work) if we want to remain free of cardiovascular disease. Meanwhile, obesity in children is rising.

We saw already that heart disease at the level of the artery doesn't start with deposits of plaque; it starts with free radical injury to the lining of the artery. It is *after* the free radical injury to the lining of the artery that your body initiates the healing response with the deposition of plaque. Eating more than your caloric demands forces the body to metabolize fuel that it doesn't need, which it stores as fat. This metabolic process causes the accumulation of excess free radicals. We looked earlier at evidence suggesting that consuming slightly fewer calories than we need may actually increase our life expectancy.

Exercise—not too much, not too little—thwarts free radical injury. Just as there's a diet tailored for free radical protection, there's a workout routine that maximizes your benefits and minimizes your free radical load. I myself am a conscientiously fit person who exercises regularly in a non-injurious way. However, when it comes to offering advice on this subject, I prefer to turn to the experts. I've therefore called on two well-known and respected professional trainers to share their wisdom with you. I have used a combination of their techniques to craft my own exercise regimen.

Bruce Krahn, author of *The Fat-Fighter Diet*, is a highly fit and knowledgeable trainer. His expertise is the area of body building and he is part of a new school of thought that promotes efficiency while protecting the body from injury. Teresa Tapp, author of *Fit and Fabulous in 15 Minutes*, is just as fit and just as knowledgeable. She offers advice on losing weight and gaining strength while respecting posture and spinal alignment. She promotes a new injury-free exercise routine designed to help us lose fat, increase health and reduce our free radical burden. Both of them have agreed to offer up an exercise program to complement *The Antioxidant Prescription*.

Bruce Krahn:
YOUR PERSONAL LOW-INJURY ANTIOXIDANT EXERCISE PLAN

In today's health-minded era, the question is no longer *if* you should exercise but, rather, *how* you should exercise. With a world full of late-night infomercials hawking everything from abdominal rollers to "gazelles," it's no wonder that many people throw up their hands in utter confusion.

Let's examine what fitness really means and then look at what we can do today to start you on your way to a healthier, more energetic life. Fitness can be described as the development of all the body's physical capabilities, including the following:

- Aerobic conditioning or "cardio." This is any activity that utilizes a large amount of oxygen, delivered to the muscles by the lungs, heart and circulatory system. Aerobic conditioning may be achieved through activities such as running, sprinting, cycling, skiing and jumping rope.
- Muscular conditioning. Resistance or weight training is the single best method to develop and strengthen the muscles. This is done by working the muscles through a full range of motion with a focus on both the eccentric (lowering) and concentric (raising) portions of a given movement.
- Flexibility. Stretching the muscles, tendons and ligaments surrounding the joints of your body will promote increased range of motion, decrease the chance of injury and improve recovery between workouts.

A well-balanced exercise regimen must include all three components in order to produce the maximum benefit.

COMPONENT #1: AEROBIC CONDITIONING

If you are like most of my clients, one of your main goals is to burn body fat and increase your energy level. In order to accomplish this, resistance training and stretching are not enough. The secret to shedding unwanted body fat while simultaneously improving heart and lung capacity lies in cardiovascular exercise. Contrary to popular belief, due to the body's starvation response, cutting calories is not the best way to burn body fat. Although it is important to eat fewer "empty" calories, it is far better for your health, energy and fitness to consume sufficient amounts of nutritious foods and exercise your way to a healthier, leaner physique.

How Much and How Often

One of the key points to remember is that *all* exercise is a form of stress on the body and that oxidative stress increases with exercise intensity and duration. Too much exercise can be harmful to the body. This is why it is important to *periodize* your training program, that is, divide your exercise program (cardio and strength) into phases of low, medium and high intensity to allow for maximum recovery and results.

What Is the Right Amount of Cardio?

The right amount of cardio for you will depend on your goal and, as Bryce Wylde writes, on the results of your latest free radical test.

If your goal is to develop a healthy lifestyle, improve your overall health, increase heart and lung capacity and lose some body fat, 20 to 30 minutes 2 or 3 times per week would be great.

If your goal is to lose body fat, I would recommend increasing this slightly to 30 or 40 minutes, 3 to 5 days per week (30 minutes if you are performing cardio on an empty stomach immediately upon waking, and 40 minutes if done any other time).

Target Heart Rate

Performing your cardio using the correct target heart rate (THR) for your body is important to your success. You can calculate your THR as follows: **220 minus your age minus resting heart rate (RHR) multiplied by intensity per cent plus your RHR.**

Your intensity level depends on your level of exercise experience. A beginner operates at an average of 50 to 65 per cent intensity, an intermediate at 65 to 80 per cent intensity and an advanced at 80 to 90 per cent intensity.

Here's an example. Let's say you're forty and new to regular workouts—in other words, you're a beginner. When you're still in bed in the morning, count your pulse for exactly 60 seconds at your wrist or at your jaw just below your ear, or wherever you can feel the beat of your heart. Let's say you find your pulse to be, on average and over 3 days, 70 beats a minute—that's your resting heart rate (RHR). These three figures—your age, your exercise status and your RHR—are all you need. Now get out a piece of paper and subtract your age (40) from 220. You get 180, which is your maximum heart rate. Now from your maximum heart rate subtract your RHR (70) to get your heart rate reserve. You get 110. Now multiply your heart rate reserve (110) by your intensity percentage (about 60 per cent, since you're a beginner) to get 66, and add to that your resting heart rate (70) to get 133, your target heart rate.

While exercising, you can check your heart rate using a strap-on heart monitor. Or you can check your pulse, counting beats for 10 seconds and multiplying that number by 6. If neither of these fairly accurate approaches suits you, you can use "conversational pace" to monitor moderate activities such as walking. If you can talk and walk at the same time, you probably aren't working too hard. But if you can sing and maintain your level of effort, you definitely aren't working hard enough. If you start puffing soon after starting or have to stop and catch your breath, you're probably going at it too hard.

Change Is Good

Performing your cardiovascular exercise in your target heart rate zone will produce excellent results. However, like resistance training, the duration, type, intensity and frequency of your cardiovascular workouts must change every couple of weeks in order to avoid your body's inevitable adaptation response. The following are some changes to consider:

1. Substitute one form of cardiovascular exercise for another, for example, stair climbing for running or sprinting for jogging.
2. Vary the duration of your cardio workout. If you have been doing 20 minutes, try 30.
3. Change the frequency of your cardiovascular workouts. Instead of 2 times per week try 3.
4. Try performing your cardio at a different intensity level.

COMPONENT #2: MUSCULAR CONDITIONING

Today's modern fitness facilities are typically filled with row after row of shiny machines. Although these machines can be useful, they simply are not necessary. All you need to enjoy an effective workout is a set of dumb-bells (2.5–15 kg [5–30 lb.]) and a stability ball.

There are four basic human movements: lunge, squat, push/pull and rotation. In order to have a well-balanced body, each of these movement patterns should be addressed within your workout program. Although there are literally thousands of exercises and even more possible routines, the following is an introduction to *resistance training*. This is an excellent start-ing point for those looking to improve their health without overtraining. Overtraining is important to avoid due to the resulting physical injury, free radical damage and decrease in immune function.

Before you begin a new exercise regimen, it is important that you com-plete the following Physical Activity Readiness Questionnaire (PAR-Q). If you are between the ages of fifteen and sixty-nine, this test will tell you if you should check with your doctor before you start exercising. If you are over sixty-nine years of age and you are not accustomed to being very active, check with your doctor.

Please read these questions carefully and answer each one honestly with yes or no.

1. Has your doctor ever said that you have a heart condition and that you should only do physical activity recommended by a doctor?

2. Do you feel pain in your chest when you do physical activity? In the past month, have you had chest pain when you were not doing physical activity?

3. Do you lose your balance because of dizziness or do you ever lose consciousness?

4. Do you have a bone or joint problem (for example, a back, knee or hip problem) that could be made worse by a change in your physical activity?

5. Is your doctor currently prescribing drugs (e.g., water pills) for your blood pressure or heart condition?

6. Do you know of any other reason why you should not do physical activity?

If you answered yes to one or more questions, talk to your doctor before you start becoming much more physically active or before you complete the fitness testing. Tell your doctor about this questionnaire and which questions you answered yes to.

If you answered no to *all* questions, you can be reasonably sure that you can take part in the following fitness testing and start becoming more physically active. I recommend, however, that you have your blood pressure tested. If you have a reading over 144/94, talk with your doctor before you start any fitness program.

The following is a beginner level / first-phase introduction to resistance training. This program should be followed for approximately 6 weeks before moving on to a different phase. Following a phase-based form of training is important in order to avoid overtraining and hitting a plateau.

FIRST-PHASE INTRODUCTION TO RESISTANCE TRAINING

BODY PART	EXERCISES	WORKOUT Sets	Rep	INTENSITY	TEMPO	REST INTERVAL
Core 1	Pelvic tilt	1–2	5	Body weight*	5-1-5	60 sec.
Core 2	Side plank (knees)	1–2	5	Body weight	Hold 30–60 sec.	60 sec.
Core 3	Front plank (knees)	1–2	n/a	Body weight	Hold 30–60 sec.	60 sec.
Thigh (Quads)	Ball squat	1–2	12–15	Body weight	3-1-1	60 sec.
Core 4	Quadruped (knees)	1–2	8 per side	Body weight	5-1-5	60 sec.
Chest	Kneeling push-up	1–2	12–15	Body weight	3-1-1	60 sec.
Back 1	One-arm dumbbell row (with ball)	1–2	12–15	65–70%	3-1-1	60 sec.
Back 2	Dumbbell pullover (lying on ball)	1–2	12–15	65–70%	3-1-1	60 sec.
Shoulders	Dumbbell shoulder press (seated on ball)	1–2	12–15	65–70%	3-1-1	60 sec.
Biceps	Dumbbell curl (seated on ball)	1–2	12–15	65–70%	3-1-1	60 sec.
Triceps	Dumbbell triceps extension (on ball)	1–2	12–15	65–70%	3-1-1	60 sec.
Abdominals	Crunch (on ball)	1–2	12–15	Body weight	3-3-3	60 sec.

*Bodyweight = without use of dumbbells; N/A = not applicable

Definition of Fitness Training Terms

1. Intensity: Defined as a percentage of your one repetition maximum (RM) for a given exercise (1 RM = 100% intensity; 5 RM = 50% intensity, etc.).

2. Tempo: The speed of each repetition. The first digit is the lowering (negative) portion in seconds, the middle digit is the pause and the third digit is the return (positive) movement.

3. Rest Interval: The length of rest time in seconds taken between sets of an exercise.

EXERCISE DESCRIPTIONS

CORE

Exercise: **Pelvic tilt.**

Starting Point: Lie on your back with knees bent, feet flat on floor, arms resting up over head. Activate core by pulling lower abdominal region inwards towards spine.

Movement: Pull lower abdominal region inwards towards your spine. Perform a slight posterior pelvic tilt by flattening lower back against floor. Hold for recommended time.

Key Points: Maintain core activation. Do not let neck hyperextend or chin jut forward. Upper body should remain motionless.

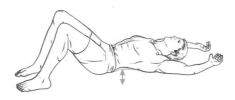

Exercise: **Side plank** (knees).

Starting Point: Lie on side with knees bent. Activate core (pull lower abdominal region in towards spine and squeeze gluteus). Place elbow directly under shoulder for support.

Movement: Maintain core activation, lift body up onto forearm and hold for recommended time. Repeat for opposite side.

Key Points: Head must stay in neutral position. Core must be activated for duration of exercise.

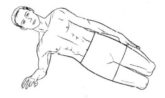

Exercise: **Front plank**
(knees).

Starting Point: Starting in a prone position, elbows bent and closed fists positioned under shoulders. Activate core (pull lower abdominal region inwards towards spine).

Movement: Lift body up onto forearms and knees. Maintain core activation and hold for recommended time.

Key Points: Spine should maintain neutral position at all times. Gluteus should remain activated throughout duration of exercise. Keep chin tucked in.

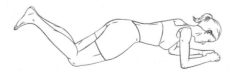

Exercise: **Quadruped** (knees).

Starting Point: Start on your hands and knees. Activate core (pull lower abdominal region inwards towards spine).

Movement: Slowly lift one arm (put thumb up) and the opposite leg until they are both straight and parallel with the floor. Hold for recommended time, then slowly lower limbs to the floor while keeping your core activated. Repeat on the opposite side.

Key Points: Maintain core activation and proper posture alignment. Think of lengthening body as you raise arm and leg rather than simply lifting.

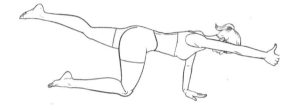

THIGH

Exercise: **Ball squat.**

Starting Point: Place a stability ball against wall. Stand with feet pointing straight ahead and gently lean back against ball so that lumbar curve is supported by the ball. Activate core (pull lower abdominal region inwards towards spine).

Movement: Maintaining core stability, descend slowly to parallel by bending at knees and hips. Return to starting position by driving through the feet and extending through ankle, knee and hip joints while maintaining equal weight distribution on both feet.

Key Points: Maintain core stability, and knees should track over second and third toe.

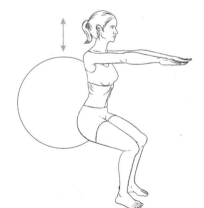

CHEST

Exercise: **Kneeling push-up.**

Starting Point: Facing the floor with your hands beside your chest as shown, in a kneeling position. Activate your core.

Movement: With your core remaining active, push up until your arms are straight then slowly lower yourself till you hover just above the floor.

Key Points: Do not lock your elbows or allow your head to jut forward. Maintain your core stability.

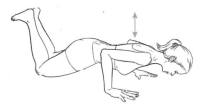

BACK

Exercise: **One-arm dumbbell row** (with ball).

Starting Point: Assume a 45-degree bent-over position with one arm extended resting on ball for support. Hold dumbbell with opposite arm hanging perpendicular to floor. Activate core (pull lower abdominal region inwards towards spine).

Movement: Maintaining optimal posture, pull dumbbell into side of chest. Slowly lower to start position and repeat for recommended repetitions.

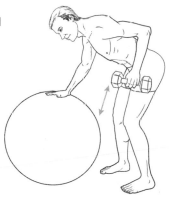

Key Points: Maintain core stability. Focus on generating movement from back—not arms.

Exercise: **Dumbbell pullover** (lying on ball).

Starting Point: Lie on back on ball with head and neck supported and hips up in line with knees and shoulders. Hold one dumbbell in both hands over chest. Activate core by pulling lower abdominal region inwards towards spine.

Movement: Maintaining optimal posture, slowly lower dumbbell backwards until dumbbell is in line with head. Using back muscles, pull dumbbell back to start position. Repeat for recommended repetitions.

Key Points: Maintain your core stability and focus the movement through your back, not your arms, keep both arms straight throughout the movement.

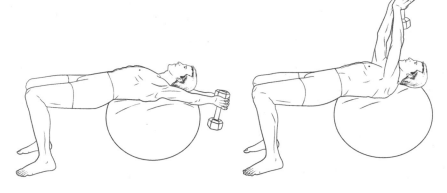

SHOULDERS

Exercise: **Dumbbell shoulder press** (seated on ball).

Starting Point: Sit on an exercise ball. Activate core (pull lower abdominals inwards towards spine). Hold dumbbells in each hand at slightly higher than shoulder height.

Movement: Maintaining core position, slowly press dumbbells upwards and together overhead. Slowly lower to start position. Repeat for recommended repetitions.

Key Points: Maintain core stability. Do not let head jut forward. Look straight ahead.

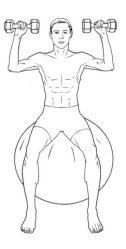

BICEPS

Exercise: **Dumbbell curl** (seated on ball).

Starting Point: Sit on ball. Hold a dumbbell in each hand with palms forward, arms extended. Activate core (pull lower abdominal region inwards towards spine).

Movement: Perform dumbbell curl by flexing elbows while keeping shoulder blades retracted. Slowly lower back to original position by extending elbows. Complete for recommended repetitions.

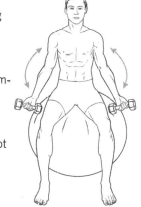

Key Points: Maintain core stability. Look straight ahead—do not jut chin forward. Pivot from elbow and keep elbow stationary.

TRICEPS

Exercise: **Dumbbell triceps extension** (on ball).

Starting Point: Lie face up on ball. Grip 2 dumbbells with hands 30 cm (12 in.) apart. Activate core (pull lower abdominal region inwards towards spine).

Movement: Slowly lower dumbbells to just slightly above forehead. Extend arm, returning to starting position. Repeat for recommended repetitions.

Key Points: Maintain core activation. Keep upper arm in vertical position

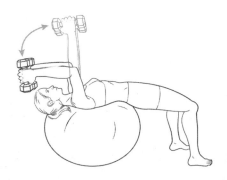

ABDOMINALS

Exercise: **Crunch** (on ball).

Starting Point: Sit on ball. Activate core by pulling lower abdominal region towards spine and squeezing gluteus. Slowly walk feet out and lie back on ball. Head and shoulders should be supported on ball with head slightly tilted back.

Movement: Slowly curl spine upwards as far as you can comfortably maintain control.

Key Points: Chin should be tucked towards chest throughout the movement. Core activation should be maintained for duration of exercise.

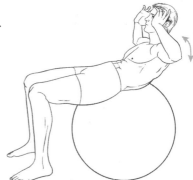

COMPONENT #3: FLEXIBILITY

Flexibility is perhaps the most neglected component of the average person's workout. The stretching of your muscles, tendons, ligaments and joint structures is vital for promoting and improving range of motion and will also result in improving the overall aesthetics of your body. Additional benefits of engaging in daily stretching include increased physical performance, decreased chance of injury, improved posture and reduced muscle soreness, increased blood flow and an improved sense of well-being. Be sure to stretch lightly before each workout (cardio and strength training). A more aggressive stretch should be completed in the postworkout period immediately following each training session.

The preceding workouts are a brief introduction to periodizing an exercise program. Changing your resistance training program on a regularly scheduled basis will ensure that your body receives the correct balance of variety, volume and intensity of work while incorporating sufficient time for recovery. If you wish to obtain a full year of periodized, phase-based training, I invite you to log on to my website at www.ebodi.com.

Teresa Tapp:
THE WELLNESS WORKOUT THAT WORKS ANYTIME, ANYWHERE

Instead of approaching exercise from the traditional perspective—calorie expenditure, aerobic conditioning and building muscle to improve body mass index—why not create full-fibre muscle activation and move your body in a special way to expand its ability to also improve physiological function and left brain–right brain mind–body balance?

I have created a preventative wellness/fitness program designed to help the body help itself repair and rebuild from the inside out, which I call T-Tapp (for more information, visit www.t-tapp.com). It is more than just another workout. Its sequence of comprehensive, compound-muscle activation, combined with leverage isometric (you against gravity) during large-muscle movement, maximizes biomechanics and improves muscle imbalance. T-Tapp helps to improve body alignment, joint health, neuro-kinetic (mind-to-muscle) transmission, circulation and lymphatic flow. By combining this type of muscle activation with linear alignment and lymphatic pumping, T-Tapp also provides cardiac conditioning without impact and promotes bone density without weights or stretchy bands. In simple terms, T-Tapp helps your body maximize muscle movement so it can receive more benefit in less time. Its optimization of lymphatic function also helps the body decrease inflammation and eliminate cellular toxicity. This is why T-Tapp works well for those who have inflammation issues such as arthritis, fibromyalgia, chronic fatigue syndrome and multiple sclerosis and, in fact, as described in this book, all free radical–induced disease.

My program's intricate design of sustained muscle resistance provides continual challenge. You never have to do more than eight repetitions and only one set of each exercise and, amazingly, as you become stronger, the workout becomes more challenging. That's hard to believe, since traditional exercise has taught us that the stronger we get the more weight and/or repetitions we must add to increase challenge and strength. But it's true. Every exercise uses the full-fibre activation of multiple muscles on all joints to increase their range of rotation during movement. For this reason, T-Tapp is safe and effective for all ages and all fitness levels and will continue to challenge you as long as you execute each exercise to your best ability.

In addition to being an all-in-one workout that builds heart health, bone density and muscles that are equally strong and flexible, T-Tapp is also an educational program that explains how to increase muscle activation with any type of exercise or activity. Using my techniques enables you to "exercise" anytime or anywhere while you sit, walk, work or play.

Is it really possible to target and tone "saddlebags" while you stand in line? Can you flatten your stomach, trim your thighs and lift your derrière while sitting? The short answer is yes.

Understanding how to activate your muscles and move your body to increase efficiency and effectiveness is the secret to success in building a body that looks and feels better. Most people report more energy, less pain and better health and lose one or two clothing sizes in four weeks of doing the workout featured in my book, *Fit and Fabulous in 15 Minutes*. Start today, while you're reading this book.

Body Alignment

Maintaining correct body alignment during movement is a primary principle. Poor posture can impair neurokinetic transmission, create muscle imbalance and alter metabolic function. Take a look at any anatomy or physiology textbook, and you'll see that the human body is positioned with arms at the sides and palms facing forward. This is considered correct anatomical position. Look at your own stance in a mirror. Are your palms facing backwards? Most people's do, but this type of stance can be problematic because it causes your shoulder joint to roll forward, which ultimately creates muscle imbalance along your upper spine.

Over time this posture can create muscle atrophy and cause your upper spine to curve forward, decrease bone health and increase fat storage at the base of your neck. Poor posture creates joint pronation in hips, knees and ankles with muscle imbalance in your lower body as well. So put your body into alignment with my recommended stance before you start the Wellness Workout and maintain the stance with every exercise.

The T-Tapp Stance

Step 1   Stand with your feet hip-width apart. Make sure that your ankles, knees and hip joints are in alignment with your toes pointed forward, not turned out.

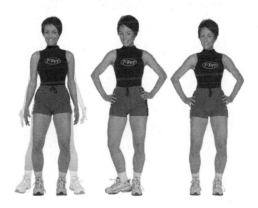

Step 2   Bend your knees. Feel how your muscles tighten just above the knees? Now straighten your knees. Feel how your thighs relax? Keep your knees slightly bent at all times.

Step 3   Tuck your butt. This is more than just tightening the gluteal muscles. Curl your butt under and press your belly button to your spine. This is similar to how a dog tucks its tail between its legs when reprimanded. Feel how your lower back and stomach muscles tighten?

Step 4   Lift your ribs and bring your shoulders back in alignment with your hips. Feel how your stomach pulled in when you lifted your rib cage? Keeping ribs up with shoulders back creates more room in your abdominal area and increased core muscle activation.

Step 5   Push knees out towards your little toe. Feel how your lower tummy tightens as well as your thighs, outer hips and butt? Feel how the arches in your feet lift? Knee-to-little-toe (KLT) position maximizes muscle activation in your lower body and provides rehabilitative benefits. Just push your knees out to the best of your ability. Then once you have built enough strength and flexibility, also press the ball joint in your foot down and lift your big toe. This will increase the intensity and stabilize your ankles.

Shoulder Rolls

Now that your body is in alignment, let's focus on your shoulders. Flip your palms forward, stretch your fingers wide, and twist your thumbs towards the wall behind you as far as you can. Feel how every muscle in your upper back tightened? Now inhale big and exhale bigger. Feel how all

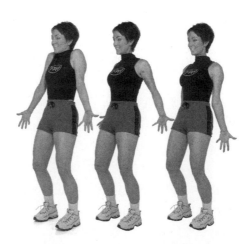

your back muscles and the muscles between your ribs achieved a deeper stretch during the inhale? Repeat, but this time when you exhale pull your shoulders down and tighten all the muscles between your ribs. Every time you inhale/exhale, try to achieve full extension and full contraction. This not only helps improve oxygenation and lymphatic flow, it can also create greater loss of inches in your torso.

Now roll your shoulders up, back and down four times, keeping your hands below your waist and your thumbs back as far as you can. Reverse with four shoulder rolls forward then finish with one more set of four shoulders rolls back.

Spine Rollup

Bend over and place your hands on the outside of your calves (not your ankles). Relax your upper body and keep your knees bent in KLT position. Inhale and exhale as you let gravitational pull release tension in your neck, shoulders and lower back. Now tighten your butt. Feel your hamstrings tighten and stretch? Then push your hands into your calves and at the same time push your knees out. Feel how you activated all your back muscles?

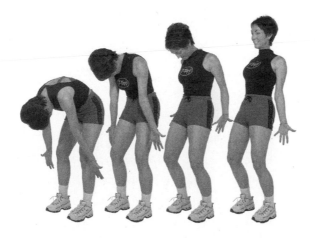

Now pull your shoulders back to create even greater activation.

Leverage isometric activation is another primary principle of my exercise program. The action of pushing into your body creates greater isometric activation and helps you maintain it longer, as well as stabilizing your spine.

Repeat inhale and exhale. Now gently rock your head four times without any other body movement.

While pushing in to maintain isometric activation, tuck your butt and slowly curl your back until your arms are straight. Then flip your palms forward, tuck more and reach your hands down with extended fingers while you continue to roll up. You should feel an extra stretch in your mid- to lower back. While rolling up one vertebra at a time, keep your hands in alignment with your shoulders by dragging your little fingers along the sides of your thigh. Don't lift your chin until your ribs are up. Finish with two shoulder rolls back.

Repeat spine rollup once more to completely warm up your spine.

Butterfly Squats

Form Check. Try to maintain squat position at all times and do all three parts without stopping.

Part 1. Place your feet shoulder-width apart, with your toes turned out at a 30-degree angle or less. Bend your knees, tuck your butt and pull your shoulders back in alignment with your hips. Maintain this position and push your knees out while you lower your body, keeping your knees in alignment with your ankles. Then extend your arms at shoulder level with palms up and thumbs back as far as you can.

Now, without bending your elbows, move your arms up and down approximately 15 cm (6 in.) for a total of 8 repetitions (1 count each).

Form Check: Reach away with your hands as if someone is pulling on your arms. When doing this, you should feel greater muscle activation, not only in your arms, but also in your shoulders and upper back. Keep your lower body actively isolated with your butt tucked and your knees pushing out at all times.

Part 2. Bend your knees a little deeper, tuck your butt a bit harder and keep your shoulders back as your increase your arm movement (shoulder to waist) for a total of 8 repetitions (2 counts each).

Form Check: Tighten your lats to stabilize your arm movement to stop at shoulder height without momentum.

Part 3. Bend your knees even deeper, tuck a little more, and lean back a little bit as you continue to lower your arms all the way down until your hands are beside your body (counts 1–2) and back up until they are level with your shoulders (counts 3–4), for a total of 8 repetions (4 counts each).

Form Check: Lift your ribs and pull your shoulders back each time you lower your arms to the sides of your body. Don't forget—always keep your thumbs back as far as you can. Repeat for a total of 8 repetitions (4 counts each). Shake out your arms and legs and take a water break.

Tip: Water breaks are important not only to hydrate your body and optimize metabolic function, but also to assist lymphatic elimination of cellular toxicity.

T-Tapp Twist Stretch

Now that lymphatic circulation has been stimulated from the butterfly squat sequence, twisting your upper body while maintaining isometric stabilization of your lower body will optimize it even more by targeting your thoracic duct, the largest lymphatic vessel in the body. This exercise is very effective at trimming your torso too!

Resume the T-Tapp stance, focusing hard on keeping your butt tucked and your knees pushing out to stabilize your hips and protect your lower back. Now place your hands just below your collarbone, with elbows level and one hand on top of the other. Then lift your ribs and pull your shoulders back and down, and press your hands together. Feel the difference? It's important to establish isometric activation in your upper back and shoulder muscles too.

Form Check: Never, ever release your butt tuck!

Inhale big and push your left knee out even more while you exhale deeply and reach back with your right elbow as far as you can and hold (counts 1–4). Then relax and release your twist but do not lower your right elbow or release your T-Tapp stance (counts 5–8). Repeat, but this time focus on pulling your ribs together, and look back at your right elbow as best you can during the exhale (counts 1–4). Then without releasing twist position, inhale bigger (counts 5–6) and exhale bigger (counts 7–8) while tucking, pushing KLT and reaching back to maximize your spinal stretch and lymphatic flow.

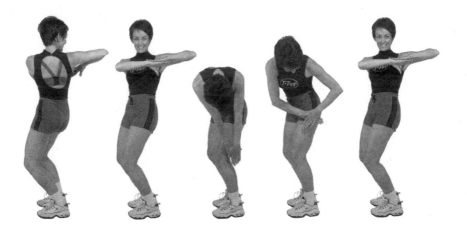

Relax and return your upper body to the starting position. Do 2 shoulder rolls back with your palms forward.

Form Check: Never allow your reaching elbow to drop lower than your shoulder.

Do 1 spine rollup, then repeat the twist stretch to the left side.

Finish with another spine rollup. Take a water break and proceed to hoe downs.

Hoe Downs

Part 1. Assume the T-Tapp stance but shift your weight to your left leg. Keep your left knee bent in KLT position, your butt tucked and your ribs up while you extend your hands out to the sides of your body with palms up and thumbs back. Your elbows should be close to your body in alignment with your shoulders, and your wrists should be level with your elbows. Now push your elbows forward and pull your hands back to your best ability. Feel every muscle in your back activate?

Inhale and exhale. Ready? Begin: Lift your right knee up in alignment with your right shoulder (count 1), and then tap your toes to the floor (count 2). Repeat for a total of 4 lifts and taps (8 counts).

Form Check: Try not to move your upper body when lifting your knee. Keep your butt tucked and your left knee bent in KLT at all times. Proceed to Part 2 without stopping.

Part 2. Lift your right knee up and out to the right side as you bring your right hand across your body to the left (count 1) and tap your toes on the floor (count 2). Repeat for a total of 4 lifts and taps (8 counts).

Form Check: Linear alignment is important during lifts and taps. In addition to aiming your knee towards the shoulder while lifting, also keep your foot pointed and in alignment with your knee.

Tip: Pointing your toe intensifies activation of abdominal muscles.

Repeat Parts 1 and 2 as follows:

Two sets of 4 lifts and taps (8 counts front, 8 counts on right side, twice); 2 sets of 2 lifts and taps (counts 1–4 front, counts 5–8 right side, twice); and 1 set of 4 single lifts and taps (counts 1–2 front, counts 3–4 right side, 4 times)—all without stopping.

Then, while inhaling and exhaling, do 1 shoulder roll back and reset starting position to repeat the same sequence on other side (2 sets of 4, 2 sets of 2, and 1 set of 4 single lifts and taps with left knee).

Then repeat the entire sequence (right side, then left side) for a total of 2 sets of hoe downs. Take a water break. (A demonstration of Hoe Downs, as well as Butterfly Squats and the T-Tapp Twist Stretch, are available as free downloads on my website, www.t-tapp.com)

Isn't it amazing how much your heart rate increases without jumping or putting your hands above your head? Isn't it amazing how much you can feel your muscles work with only 8 repetitions? Visible results can be seen within days because T-Tapp exercises build muscles with density instead of traditional isotonic mass. This type of muscle development empowers your muscles to work like spandex to uplift, cinch, tighten and tone quicker.

ANTIOXIDANT SUPPLEMENTS TAILORED FOR EXERCISE: THE AMINO ACID TRIAD

I've long admired Bruce Krahn and Teresa Tapp, not only for their disciplined and informed approach to the challenge of fitness, but also because their work so closely dovetails with my own and modern integrative medicine's interest in reducing stress—physical stress in this case—and reducing free radical burden. To their wisdom, I'd now like to add a little of my own.

Certain amino acids have the remarkable ability to act as exercise enhancers. On days when you're exercising, these supplements will promote fat loss, muscle gain and a reduction in the overall free radical burden from exercise.

Amino acids are derived from protein and act as building blocks in the body. Some have the capacity to act as free radical scavengers too. They're highly effective at therapeutic ranges. But you should exercise caution. Given their sheer effectiveness, you'll want to discuss appropriate quantities with a qualified health-care practitioner. Some amino acids can control blood sugar levels, a positive thing for most, but perhaps not for a diabetic who is already taking controlling medications. Some can thin the blood or reduce blood pressure, again, a nice benefit for some people but not for those on certain heart medications. Overall, however, the three amino acids I recommend—I call them the "Amino Acid Triad"—can enhance slimming, enhance oxygen exchange, lower free radical damage and make astonishing improvements to your overall fitness level.

L-Carnitine

The body manufactures L-carnitine from the amino acids lycine and methionine to release energy from stored fat. It transports fatty acids into mitochondria—those little powerhouses within each one of our trillions of cells. Besides being an exercise enhancer and an antioxidant, L-carnitine also appears to play an important role for the heart. As an example, patients with diabetes and high blood pressure were given 4 g of L-carnitine per day in a preliminary study. After 45 weeks, irregular heartbeat and abnormal heart functioning were improved significantly compared with non-supplemented patients. For congestive heart failure, much of the research has used a modified form of carnitine called propionyl-L-carnitine (PC). In one double-blind trial, using 500 mg PC per day led to a 26 per cent increase in exercise capacity after six months. In other research, patients with congestive heart failure given 1.5 g PC daily for 15 days experienced a 21 per cent increase in exercise tolerance and a 45 per cent increase in oxygen consumption. Research also shows that people who supplement with L-carnitine while engaging in an exercise regimen are less likely to experience muscle soreness from the buildup of lactic acid.

For general fitness enhancement and "leaning up," I recommend about 10 mg of L-carnitine per .5 kg (1 lb.) of body weight, taken on an empty stomach twice daily (especially important on those days of exercise). An empty stomach for optimal absorption of amino acids means 30 minutes before eating or 90 minutes after mealtime.

L-Arginine

This amino acid is of particular interest to me due to its roles in the cardiovascular system. It plays several roles in addition to acting as a free radical scavenger, but paradoxically, in excess, it can cause an elevation of nitric oxide to the point that free radical damage ensues, so be careful not to exceed the recommended doses of this one. As a precursor to nitric oxide, which the body uses to keep blood vessels dilated, it allows the heart to receive adequate oxygen and researchers have begun to use arginine in people with angina and congestive heart failure. New time-released formulas are becoming available. Arginine also appears to act as a natural blood thinner, and other evidence suggests that it may even help regulate cholesterol levels. However, if you have already experienced a heart attack, avoid L-arginine.

Its roles in the body include assistance in wound healing (at 17 g per day), in removing excess ammonia from the body, in stimulating immune function and in promoting secretion of several hormones, including glucagon, insulin and growth hormone. Incidentally, we've been trying to reach our broker, Will Powers, to tell him to stay away from L-arginine, which antagonizes herpes virus, the cause of cold sores. Of course, when we last heard from Will, he'd deserted his buddy's yacht, *Free Radical,* and had little interest in looking after his health. Still, we can hope.

But it's the effect of arginine on growth hormone levels that has interested bodybuilders and fitness gurus alike. In a controlled trial, when arginine and ornithine (500 mg of each, twice per day, 5 times per week) were combined with weight training, a greater decrease in body fat was obtained after only 5 weeks than when the same exercise was combined with a placebo.

For general energy, vitality and cardiovascular support, I recommend about 10 mg per .5 kg (1 lb.) of body weight, taken on an empty stomach twice daily morning and evening and at least at 30 minutes apart from L-carnitine.

L-Glutamine

Glutamine is the most abundant amino acid in the body and is involved in more metabolic processes than any other amino acid. The amino acid glutamine appears to play a role in several aspects of human physiology that might benefit athletes, including their muscle function and immune system. Double-blind trials giving athletes glutamine (5 g after intense, prolonged exercise, then again 2 hours later) reported 81 per cent having improved immune function.

It is my recommendation to consider L-glutamine along with the other two amino acids, in part because intense exercise lowers blood levels of glutamine, which can remain persistently low when regularly training. Glutamine supplementation may raise natural levels of growth hormone at an intake of 2 g per day, an effect of interest to some athletes because of the role of growth hormone in stimulating muscle growth, and glutamine, given intravenously, was found to be more effective than other amino acids at helping replenish muscle glycogen after exercise. Lastly, glutamine (especially the C-glutamine form) also serves as a source of fuel for cells lining the intestines. I often use this with my patients when working on the third R—regeneration—of the 4 Rs. Without it, intestinal cells can waste away.

For general fitness enhancement and immune support, I recommend about 40 mg of C-glutamine (or L-Glutamine) per .5 kg (1 lb.) of body weight twice daily on an empty stomach, between meals and away from the other amino acids.

EXERCISE: SOME FINAL THOUGHTS

There has been no pill invented that can replace the need to exercise, but if one existed, it would contain these three amino acids and the nutrients we looked at in the previous chapter. And my strong feeling is that if everyone exercised as much as they should, upwards of 90 per cent of all known chronic disease would be prevented or managed effectively.

Meanwhile, the not-so-traditional yet methodical exercise suggestions offered by Bruce Krahn point to an effective way to whip ourselves into shape while protecting ourselves from injury. And Teresa Tapp offers a new look at exercise physiology, a unique approach to keeping fit and a way to accomplish these goals no matter where we find ourselves or whatever the time constraints.

No, a miracle exercise pill doesn't exist. But I offer the information in this book as a fair substitute.

CHAPTER 12

A LIFE WORTH LIVING

S o you've got a crazy cousin, Emily. She's allergic to every-thing, is a total vegan and manages to corner you at every family gathering and lecture you about vitamin C—*lots* of vitamin C. Hoo boy. Amazing you even *looked* at this book, but you have. Now what?

Although growing up vegetarian and unvaccinated was my experience, I can't say for sure that either was the *right* thing. In fact, I'm no longer vegetarian, and with respect to vaccinations, I remain on the fence—with just as much good to say about them as bad.

But my two-year-old got a gluten-free, fructose-instead-of-sugar, preservative-free carob cake for his birthday and he loved it. My six-month-old has just started a daily dose of purified fish oils and antioxidants and she is extremely healthy. If we wipe our children's faces with chemical-free soaps and the little tykes often smell of tea tree oil and receive sixteen daily vitamins and minerals instead of the ten I received, I'm perfectly happy about that. The legacy of the sprout, tomato and SoyPro sandwich on thick German-style bread also survives. From my present perspective, I see I was lucky to have had a "fringe" mom who pummelled me with antioxidants. She was simply a woman ahead of her time.

I know I may have left you wondering whether you're pushing your personal health threshold, if perhaps you're in danger of boiling over, wondering what you should change to improve your prospects. Maybe you're questioning how much your genes have contributed to your present status or whether your body's burden of free radical molecules is a consequence of the stress you've always assumed was inseparable from your life. Maybe you've recently begun casting a baleful eye at your cell phone or the stew of toxic materials and chemicals that bob around in your immediate environment. Perhaps you're even considering getting tested. Perhaps your shopping cart is looking more colourful.

I didn't undertake this book to alarm you. I wrote it to empower you as a consumer and to persuade you that you have unique needs. I want you to know that you can protect yourself from illness and an untimely demise. I want you to see what happens on the molecular level, and to see for yourself what we've been ignoring for years while scientific research—not "bad" science or "fringe" science, but hard-nosed, hard-won worldwide consensus science—has been right under our noses. This journey to the truth began for me as a puzzle during those years in a student clinic when I realized that homeopathic medicines weren't working at their known potential. There was a major "obstacle to cure." Eventually I discovered that this obstacle was free radical activity in the body and the solution had been uncovered too: antioxidant therapy. But this truth has spread slowly, even within the broader scientific and medical community. After reading this book, you may understand more about free radical chemistry and its consequences than do many health professionals.

We've seen that free radicals are not free at all, in the sense that they make us pay the highest price of all: *our health*. Such seemingly benign things as plastics and the all-too-often pesticide-laden fruits and vegetables we eat to stay healthy—even these are hurting us through the mechanism of excessive oxidation. In Appendix C of this book, you can visit a food-additive cemetery where lie buried those additives that were once thought harmless. We're reminded—just as we are in human cemeteries—that there are plenty more to be "buried." Yet, like sleepwalkers—sleep*eaters*—we continue to consume these additives.

We've seen that it's not just additives, automotive emissions, industrial pollutants, cigarette smoke, x-rays and sunlight radiation that cause free radicals. Study after study in recent decades has shown that lifestyle—emotional stress and physical trauma and deep-fried batters and sugary, salty foods and overly strenuous exercise—all contribute heavily to their formation. As though that weren't enough, we've seen that our genes contain little mutations that become more inclined to express their unwanted characteristics as a result of the oxidative damage done by free radicals. We've seen free radicals to be involved in every disease, including those as severe as cancer and AIDS, and we've seen the role of radicals in the aging process. We've seen the army of new technologies that allow us to determine our free radical status and any damage being done to our DNA. And most astonishing and fortunate of all, we've seen how antioxidants—the right amounts and types—can play a critical role in solving this ancient and modern dilemma.

I've tried to set out a straightforward handbook that can guide you step by step to a reduction of your personal burden of free radicals. But the whole story is actually too big to fit into a single book. In my next book, I will focus on "debunking the junk" and reveal as much as I know about which antioxidants and natural medicines are worthy of your consideration. I would argue that at least 50 per cent of the bottled supplements, herbs and homeo-pathics crowding the shelves of health food stores are *garbage*. A pill of chalk is not a calcium supplement. I'm going to explain how to avoid this junk and how to find products from supple-ment companies that are willing to spend money to ensure their products meet standardized "good manufacturing practices."

Now, you might ask, what about Will Powers? You'll remember how Will allowed himself to be tempted back to work as a bro-kerage executive for no better reason than that the job paid two hundred grand a year with a whack of stock options. He said good-bye to the *Free Radical*—that was the name of the yacht—and caught a plane home from Samoa.

Within eight weeks, the guy had an outbreak of cold sores. He got over it but the virus struck again and came back regularly after that. I'm afraid Will couldn't see the writing on the, er, lip and his body took it upon itself to teach him a lesson. It was almost as though it wanted to put him out of commission to give him the chance to recoup on a deeper level. He came down with the shingles—a maddening disease manifest by painful blistering lesions all across his torso, followed by an itch equivalent to a great mass of mosquito bites all over the same area.

This was not a lesson Will found easy to learn. He was laid up in bed for weeks, but this didn't stop him from using his cell phone and laptop to do business. He'd been making half-hearted efforts to keep his fish-and-fresh-food diet going, but now decided he must order restaurant food. Meanwhile, he could hardly sleep because of the itching. He didn't know it—and wouldn't have wanted to—but he'd boiled over his health threshold. He was at about 160 per cent of his personal threshold and rising. His immune system was shot. His productivity was nil. Meanwhile, Powers had always been a single-malt man so he eased his distress with bottles of old Lagavulin and Talisker. Finally, the shingles healed and he decided he had to get himself back in shape. Will Powers took up weightlifting and started to train for a marathon. He lived on Omaha steaks to gain muscle mass and rich Caesar salads because you're supposed to eat green stuff.

Will Powers died on his way into the gym at six on a Saturday morning. He was forty-seven. A lot of people came to his funeral, but the word at the office was that things were running smoothly without him.

You think I'd end this book like that? I just wanted to see if you were awake.

Actually, it really did go something like that after Will left the yacht and came back to run the brokerage office—for about two months. It took him that long to realize he wasn't having fun. He went to talk his situation over with his homeopath. Just kidding again—Will didn't know anything about health. His good health on the boat arose from the lifestyle, not from his knowledge of free radicals. He actually went to see his financial manager.

"What's my total worth?" Will asked.

"Hm." His manager frowned. "At the moment, you're not worth much more than, say, five hundred thousand. It's going to take years to rebuild."

"How long could a guy live on that?"

The accountant frowned more deeply.

"Forever, I guess, as a pauper. You'd have no standard of living to speak of. You wouldn't even be able to pay your condo fees."

"Send me a bill for your services," said Will.

He couldn't rejoin the *Free Radical*, which had gone down off Bali, but signed on as crew aboard the graceful *DaSylva* out of Auckland. Eventually, he became her captain. But he worked moderately hard and ate well and hardly ever had a cold sore. A young woman who joined the *DaSylva* for a summer introduced him to the beauty of yoga and Will never again imagined that "tone" was all about biceps.

And one warm November night a few years later, a passenger—a functional medicine guy from Canada—filled him in on the war with the free radicals and the hidden power of the antioxidant.

Will Powers has never again worried about a merger or an approaching downturn. Storms are his only threat and he actually loves storms. "Better typhoons than tycoons," he says to the young deckhands, who always smile in a puzzled way.

Free radicals are involved in the regulation of genetic material and they are heavily implicated in cancer. They affect quality of food, function as the underlying mechanism of a toxin, determine how fast we age and the very limits of our existence. Within the next decade, antioxidant therapy will become a treatment specialty in and of itself. Some already do, but soon many hospitals will incorporate the brilliant healing powers of antioxidant therapy. Most pharmacies will allot substantial shelf space to antioxidant supplements. Most doctors will recommend antioxidants instead of drugs as their first strategy to improve their patients' health. Drugs will come later and only if necessary.

The future of antioxidant therapy holds more than just promise. Indeed, by influencing our genetic code over millions of years, antioxidants have been a primary player in the very evolution of the human race. Theories on health come and go, but the effects of free radical biology and chemistry on medicine are here to stay.

Doctors will test you for your free radical status as routinely as they now screen cholesterol levels. Antioxidants will be customized to treat specific diseases known to be caused by specific free radicals. The future will bring research facilities dedicated to further discovery of free radical biology and entire institutions will be dedicated to teaching their findings.

We've seen free radical research mature from the simple chemical depiction of oxidants and antioxidants to the recognition of these types of molecules in cell signalling and gene expression. Free radical research is destined to transform personal and even general public health. When you undertake a free radical self-test or push your doctor to test you, or adopt a personal antioxidant supplement plan or nutritional routine or exercise program of the type I've described in this book, you'll simply be incorporating the most important discovery of health sciences in the last century into your life: free radicals, at the molecular level, are *the cause of all disease.*

So continue to ignore your crazy cousin if you must. But follow just some of the recommendations I'm offering you—use this medicine of the present and the future in any way—and I'll count my efforts as successful.

Um, sesame snap, anyone?

APPENDIX A

THE ANTIOXIDANT QUIZ

Take this qualifying quiz before you read further in my book. If you score less than 10, promise yourself that you will read it right to the end. If you score between 11 and 14, you're well informed about the latest nutrition and antioxidant research, and well prepared to think about implementing my action plan. If you score 15, put the book back on the shelf and call me immediately: I want you on my team.

1. What is the best way to prepare vegetables to retain the most antioxidant activity?

    (a) Serve raw
    (b) Steam lightly
    (c) Boil
    (d) Microwave
    (e) It depends

2. Which of the following can neutralize "bad" cholesterol so it doesn't damage your arteries?

(a) Papaya
(b) Sweet potato
(c) Nuts
(d) None of the above
(e) All of the above

3. For *preventative* regimens, experts recommend getting antioxidants from food as well as relying on supplements because

(a) Supplements mostly contain therapeutic levels of antioxidants, whereas foods contain maintenance amounts.
(b) Supplements do not contain the variety of phytochemicals that fruits and vegetables do.
(c) Many people can't remember to take pills.
(d) Supplements must be taken in megadoses to have an effect.

4. Which drink bestows the most heart-healthy antioxidant power?

(a) Red wine
(b) Green tea
(c) Pomegranate juice
(d) Cranberry juice
(e) Orange juice

5. A free radical is

(a) A cell that promotes health throughout the body.

(b) A naturally or artificially occurring substance that causes disease if left unchecked.

(c) A vitamin that is distributed at no charge at health food stores and natural-medicine clinics.

(d) A nutrient that works to correct any imbalance in your body.

6. Which action causes free radicals to form, potentially putting you at greater risk of heart disease?

(a) Eating pie à la mode

(b) Breathing

(c) Taking high amounts of a single antioxidant

(d) Exercise

(e) All of the above

(f) None of the above

7. Which of the following statements is true as it relates to your genes and free radical activity in your body?

(a) Free radicals promote gene and cell division.

(b) Your DNA is unaffected by free radicals.

(c) Free radicals can cause genetic mutations.

(d) Free radicals cause cancer.

(e) Two of the above.

8. Which statement is false?

(a) In general, more colour in fruits and veggies indicates greater antioxidant activity.

(b) Consuming different coloured fruits and veggies in a meal will usually ensure a wider variety of nutrients.

(c) You should shoot for three servings of fruits and veggies a day.

(d) Eating lots of antioxidant-rich fruits and veggies will also fill you up, preventing you from overeating.

9. Which of the following does *not* contain antioxidants?

(a) Pizza

(b) Whole grains

(c) Nuts

(d) Chocolate

(e) Coffee

(f) None of the above

(g) All of the above

10. Under special circumstances, free radicals can be a *good* thing for your body because

(a) They can give you a boost of energy at the end of a long-distance workout.

(b) They are the weaponry your body uses to fight off viruses and bacteria.

(c) They can protect your skin from the sun's harmful rays.

(d) They cause mutations in our genetic code, and without that our species wouldn't evolve.

11. The following environmental toxin causes harmful amounts of free radicals to accumulate in the body:

(a) Sunlight, UV and solar radiation
(b) Cellphone-tower radiation
(c) "Background" radiation
(d) Industrial smog
(e) They all do

12. Which of the following medical investigation techniques does *not* cause free radical accumulation in the body?

(a) Medical x-rays
(b) CAT scans
(c) Mammography
(d) Ultrasound

13. Which of the following will cause the most free radical accumulation in your body?

(a) Spending four hours in a smoke-laden bar
(b) An intense two-hour workout
(c) Drinking five beers
(d) Eating two combos at McDonald's
(e) Listening to an hour-long lecture from your boss
(f) All of the above except b
(g) All of the above are approximately equal

14. Which of the following does not have antioxidant qualities?

(a) Vitamin E
(b) Vitamin K

(c) Calcium

(d) Omega-3 fatty acids

(e) All of the above

15. Which of the following drinks has the highest antioxidant activity?

(a) Black tea (no milk or sugar)

(b) Orange juice

(c) Milk

(d) Red wine

(e) Apple juice

QUIZ ANSWERS

1. The correct answer is (b): Steam lightly. Cooking vegetables over a long period of time or in large amounts of water can reduce vitamin C content, but cooking does make some antioxidants, such as lycopene in tomatoes and beta-carotene in carrots, more easily absorbed by the body. To minimize nutrient loss, steaming and stir-frying are good cooking methods. How you prepare vegetables, however, is less important than eating generous servings of a wide variety of them.

2. The correct answer is (e): All of the above. All three of these foods are rich in health-promoting antioxidants. In a health study that is still under way, researchers compared the diets of more than 73,000 nurses and found that a diet rich in vitamin E (found in nuts) reduced heart attack risk by 52 per cent, a diet rich in vitamin C (abundant in papaya) reduced risk by 43 per cent and a diet rich in beta-carotene (plentiful in sweet potatoes) reduced risk by 38 per cent. Nurses who regularly took in this trio of nutrients were 63 per cent less likely to have heart attacks than those who did not.

3. The correct answer is (b). When you snack on a carrot, for instance, you get beta-carotene as well as the countless other carotenoids found in orange and yellow fruits and veggies. Such subtle arrays of phytochemicals can't be replicated by supplements.

4. The correct answer is (c): Pomegranate juice. When it comes to antioxidant punch, pomegranate juice is off the charts. Studies show that a glass of this fruit juice packs more polyphenol antioxidants than any other drink.

5. The correct answer is (b). Because free radicals are missing an electron, they are considered unstable. Antioxidant vitamins and minerals lend electrons to these free radicals, thus neutralizing their harmful effects and protecting against conditions such as heart disease, premature aging and cancer.

6. The correct answer is (e): All of the above. Believe it or not, all of these situations can cause the formation of free radicals. Don't panic though: Everyone eats sweets from time to time, and exercise also bestows many health benefits. Breathing is a natural fact of life. The point is that if you follow a healthy diet that's chock full of antioxidants, you can mop up the free radicals, vanquishing their harmful effects.

7. The correct answer is (e): Two of the above (c and d). Free radicals can cause base pairs, the building blocks of your DNA, to switch and mutate, which then can spark the initial stages of cancer.

8. The correct answer is (c). Three is not enough, though of course it's better than nothing. Ideally, you should aim for five to nine servings of fruits and veggies daily to pack in the protection you need. According to the Dietary Guidelines for Americans, released jointly by the U.S. Department of Agriculture and the U.S. Department of Health and Human Services, children ages two to six should eat five servings of fruits and vegetables a day; children over age six, active women and teens should eat seven; and active teen boys and men should eat nine. Following a rainbow eating plan by reaching for lots of colourful produce is a powerful way to protect your heart.

9. The correct answer is (f). All of these foods contain antioxidants that can help protect your ticker (in the case of pizza, tomatoes supply the powerful nutrients). However, be sure to enjoy these foods in moderation. Pizza and chocolate contain saturated fat; nuts, which contain heart-healthy, monounsaturated fat, are still high in fat and calories and can cause weight gain. Obesity is a risk factor for heart disease.

10. The correct answer is (b). Under special circumstances free radicals can be a *good* thing for your body because, ultimately, they are the weaponry your body uses to fight off viruses and bacteria.

11. The correct answer is (e): They all do.

12. The correct answer is (d): Ultrasound.

13. The correct answer is (g): All of them are roughly equal.

14. The correct answer is (c): Calcium.

15. The correct answer is (d): Red wine.

MORE ABOUT TOXINS

PLASTICS

The potential dangers of plastics are to some degree recognized by government and industry, and plastics are categorized for recycling purposes. That's the reason for the numbers on the bottoms of bottles of water and other plastic containers. Here are the seven standard codes.

#1 PETE or PET (polyethylene terephthalate): used for most clear beverage bottles.

#2 HDPE (high-density polyethylene): used for "cloudy" milk and water jugs and opaque food bottles.

#3 PVC or V (polyvinyl chloride): used in some cling wraps (especially commercial brands) and some "soft" bottles.

#4 LDPE (low-density polyethylene): used in food storage bags and some "soft" bottles.

#5 PP (polypropylene): used in rigid containers, including some baby bottles and some cups and bowls.

#6 PS (polystyrene): used in foam "clam-shell"-type containers, meat and bakery trays and, in its rigid form, in clear takeout containers, as well as some plastic cutlery and cups.

#7 Other (usually polycarbonate): used in 5-gallon water bottles, some baby bottles, some metal can linings. Polycarbonate can release its primary building block, bisphenol A, into liquids and foods.

Not all plastic containers are labelled, but several of these categories deserve special mention.

PVC (#3) is used in food packaging, including plastic trays for boxed cookies or chocolates, candy bar wrappers and bottles. Cling wraps, including the kind used commercially to wrap meats, cheeses and other foods, are often also PVC. These and other traces of toxic chemicals, including phthalates used to soften PVC, can leach into our food, especially fatty foods at higher temperatures. The result is that we are exposed to these chemicals every day. PVC is also commonly used in teethers and soft squeeze toys for young children, beach balls, bath toys, dolls and other products such as knapsacks, raincoats and umbrellas. Again, it's the phthalates that are causing concern about the health of children playing with these soft PVC toys.

A recent study in *Environmental Health Perspectives* concluded that some styrene compounds leaching from polystyrene food containers (#6 PS) are estrogenic (meaning they can disrupt normal hormonal functioning). Worryingly, styrene is also considered a possible human carcinogen by the World Health Organization's International Agency for Research on Cancer.

Ironically, many plastics regarded as "green" or "healthy"—those used in Nalgene bottles, big water bottles used for water coolers, Brita pitchers, Avent and other baby bottles, most plastics with recycling number #7 on the bottom, the lining of tin canned foods and the various dental "sealants"—contain a chemical called bisphenol A, a potential estrogen-mimicking agent and hormone disruptor. Some studies have suggested that bisphenol A may have a negative impact on our health even at the parts-per-trillion level—the equivalent of one drop of chemical in a lake. Such a finding is alarming since most chemicals are marketed as having a safe "threshold" for consumption. The plastics industry acknowledges that leaching can take place at parts-per-billion levels—leaching of most chemicals found in plastic is more likely to take place through heating or when the container is scuffed, scratched, old or worn—but the industry disputes the claim that parts-per-trillion levels could be harmful. In 1998, the Japanese government ordered manufacturers there to recall and destroy polycarbonate tableware meant for use by children because it contained excessive amounts of bisphenol A. Health Canada announced further testing on bisphenol A—one of two hundred chemicals—in 2007, and it took the first steps towards a ban on the substance in April 2008, labeling it toxic. I think by the time this book is published, there will be moves made in North America to ban other such substances too.

AUTOMOTIVE TOXINS

By a best estimate, there are some 750,000,000 motor vehicles in the world. Who doesn't know that cars pollute? Who doesn't know that car manufacturers are supplied by steel mills that churn out hydrochloric acid, manganese compounds, finely divided metal particulates, phenol, naphthalene, benzene and the so-called greenhouse gas, carbon dioxide? Petroleum refineries process crude oil into fuels such as gasoline and diesel to run these vehicles, and they manufacture non-fuel products such as lubricating oils and asphalt, and raw materials such as benzene, toluene and xylene for the chemical industry. In the course of refining crude oil, these refineries emit toxic particulates; sulphur dioxide; nitrogen oxide; carbon monoxide; and volatile, poisonous organic compounds such as benzene, toluene, and xylene.

We're all aware that these chemical emissions cause acid rain. What is less well understood is that acid rain creates acidic soils that leach from our fruit and vegetable crops the very antioxidants, vitamins and minerals required to *protect* us from pollution. We need more antioxidants to protect us from this pollution, and the pollution itself is ensuring that we get less.

OTHER CHEMICALS
Dioxins and Furans

These persistent synthetic chemicals may be products of waste incinerators, chemical and pesticide manufacturing and pulp and paper bleaching. The World Health Organization classifies dioxins and furans as "known human carcinogens." A report released by the U.S. Environmental Protection Agency in 1994 declared that there was no safe level of dioxin. In addition to its carcinogenic potential, dioxin causes skin disorders; impairs liver, reproductive, immune and endocrine system function; and increases the incidence of miscarriages and birth defects. An estimated 90 per cent of dioxin and furan exposure is through our diet, since these chemicals are absorbed into our fat tissues—we say they're "lipophilic"—and into the fatty tissues of many animals and fish species. We know we should eat more fish to keep our hearts and immune systems healthy. But many of the most beneficial fish species are also carriers of these deadly chemicals and free radical instigators.

Polychlorinated Biphenyls (PCBs)

PCBs are commonly used in a variety of applications, from hydraulic equipment to plasticizers in paint and pigments and dyes. The World Health Organization classifies PCBs as "probable human carcinogens." PCBs, banned since 1977, continue to appear in soil, water and the atmosphere today because they mix into and bind onto anything and become ubiquitous and persistent environmental toxins. They too are lipophilic and have been proven to cause skin conditions such as acne and rashes as well as impair liver function. Studies involving animals suggest that PCBs may cause liver, stomach and thyroid gland injury; immune system changes; behavioural changes; and liver and biliary tract cancer. These studies also suggest PCBs may have a negative effect on reproduction. Infants born to mothers who consumed fish oil contaminated with PCBs were shown to have an increased incidence of impaired motor skills, a decrease in short-term memory and impaired immune function.

Pesticides

Agricultural pesticides and those used for lawns and gardens may be found in runoff that eventually flows into lakes and rivers. Pesticides cause cancer and are extremely toxic to our nervous systems. Supported by a $1.5 million grant from the U.S. Department of Defense, researchers at the Salk Institute identified a gene in 2003 that may link certain pesticides and chemical weapons to a number of neurological disorders, including Gulf War syndrome and attention-deficit/hyperactivity disorder (ADHD). This finding was one of the first to demonstrate a clear genetic link between neurological disorders and exposure to organophosphate chemicals, a group that includes household pesticides as well as deadly nerve gases such as sarin. Most arguments in favour of pesticides rested on the assumption that the exposure was minimal and the pros of consuming fruits and vegetables outweighed the cons. But this argument overlooked the effects of cumulative exposure over time and the truth revealed by recent research: our genetic makeup—and thus our health status—determines how we deal with the exposure.

Dioxins, furans, PCBs and pesticides act at the molecular and cellular level, as most free radicals do, to steal electrons from the body's molecules and blow holes in cell membranes. No good can come from these chemicals entering our bodies. Exposure to any or all of them, no matter how minimal, increases our need for antioxidants.

HEAVY METALS

Mercury, arsenic, lead and cadmium are among the metals known to have detrimental effects on humans. All are commonly released by a huge variety of industrial processes.

Mercury

"Quicksilver" is a potent neurotoxin and there is no known safe level of mercury in the human body. New research on the toxic effects of mercury on children has prompted Health Canada to advise Canadians to limit their consumption of certain fish— fresh and frozen tuna, shark, swordfish, escolar, marlin and orange roughy. Mercury toxicity is commonly associated with destruction of nervous system tissue. Women of child-bearing age should be most concerned with mercury contamination, since the mercury may be passed to the fetus, increasing the risk of learning disabilities and neurobehavioural disorders in newborns that may persist through childhood. The body unfortunately allows mercury into the brain through the blood-brain barrier, and mercury in the brain and nervous system—even in ultraminute amounts—prevents new and old nerve connections from forming. Worse, it takes the body years to clear even a small amount and it may never clear it entirely.

"Silver filling" is slang for an amalgam tooth restoration. Amalgam restorations consist of mercury, silver, tin, copper and a trace amount of zinc. Researchers have measured a daily release of mercury into the body from typical amalgam fillings that is on the order of 10 micrograms. Mercury is a toxic metal; the most minute amount damages cells. The University of Calgary's Faculty of Medicine, Department of Physiology and Biophysics, has recently provided conclusive evidence that *there is no safe level of mercury in the body.* Their findings alone will alarm you.

Mercury challenges the systemic functions of every individual and of developing fetuses, so it can lead to health problems in the average person and fetal malformations in pregnant women. Mercury leakage is most often a slow, insidious process. Health problems caused by dental mercury poisoning may emerge many years after the amalgams are replaced. Though a mercury filling may indeed be better than a rotted tooth leading to a brain infection, modern dentistry now provides safe alternatives.

Arsenic

Most familiar to us as the innocuous powder that may be slipped into your gin if you're a character in a mystery murder, arsenic is commonly associated today with groundwater contamination. It may also be found in fish and fish oil. We can distinguish chronic exposure from acute exposure by the symptoms they cause: Acute poisoning results in vomiting, esophageal and abdominal pain, and bloody diarrhea. Long-term exposure may cause skin, lung, urinary bladder and kidney cancer as well as hyperkeratoses, wart-like skin growths, which can become cancerous. We know from recent studies that arsenic acts by creating super-

oxide in cells, a very unstable free radical that is rapidly converted into hydrogen peroxide by enzymes in the cells. The
hydrogen peroxide is in turn converted into hydroxyl radicals,
which are extremely reactive and damaging free radicals that
attack cell membranes and DNA to create mutations. The mutation rate shot up still higher when researchers added a chemical
that reduced the cells' production of natural antioxidants. This
was consistent with previous research suggesting that antioxidants can protect cells from arsenic-induced genetic damage.
These studies provide some of the more recent and ever-increasing
evidence that environmental carcinogens act predominantly
through a free radical pathway.

Arsenic, by the way, is among the top environmental contaminants on the Environmental Protection Agency's "Superfund
list"—a U.S. federal government program to clean up uncontrolled hazardous waste sites.

Lead

This famously toxic metal has the potential to harm the developing brains of fetuses and children, leading to learning disabilities,
behavioural problems and mental retardation. Lead exposure
affects the nervous and reproductive systems and the kidneys and
may cause high blood pressure and anemia. Recently there has
been a widespread recall of children's toys across North America
due to lead contamination in the paint used in them. Millions of
children in Canada and the United States were needlessly exposed
to unsafe levels of lead. Part of the blame lies with toy companies
that were trying to save a buck by outsourcing production to
third-world countries, and part of the blame lies with the lack of
accountability for the sourcing of work across the globe.

The propensity for lead to catalyze free radical reactions has
been demonstrated in multiple studies. These lead-induced free

radicals inhibit the production of antioxidants, inhibit enzyme reactions, cause inflammation in cells within the artery wall, and damage DNA and inhibit its natural repair. They also initiate destruction of cellular membranes.

RADIATION
Radon
Radon is a cancer-causing radioactive gas, the product of the radioactive decay of radium within the earth. The gas normally percolates upwards and escapes into the atmosphere. But radon can easily collect in our constructed environments: our water supply, basement crawl space, brick or rock walls, slab joints, sump pump or floor drain. You cannot see it, smell it or taste it, but inhaled radon enters the lungs, where it undergoes further radioactive decay that can damage your DNA. There are no immediate symptoms. It typically takes years of exposure before a fatal lung cancer may appear. The U.S. Surgeon General has warned that radon is the second leading cause of lung cancer in the United States today. Testing for radon gas is widely available.

Solar Radiation
But if the idea of a toxic gas leaking into our basements from Mother Earth smacks of science-fiction creepiness, the truth about solar radiation (it literally does come from outer space) is even creepier! Melanoma is a highly malignant type of skin cancer that arises in melanocytes, the cells that produce pigment (skin colour). The disease can occur when ultraviolet (UV) radiation, emitted from the sun, comes in repeated, unprotected contact with your skin, especially at those vulnerable sites that have a higher density of melanocytes, such as moles and freckles. In fact, melanoma usually begins in a mole.

In a recent survey by the U.S. Centers for Disease Control, 74 per cent of young adults and 50 per cent of older adults said that they had little or no knowledge about melanoma. Startlingly, it is now the fastest-growing cancer in the United States, and by extrapolation also in Canada. In the United States, your chance of getting melanoma in 1940 was 1 in 1,500. By 2004, it was 1 in 67. By 2010, scientists predict it will be 1 in 50. There are as many new cases of melanoma each year as there are of cases of AIDS. Some 59,000 new cases of melanoma were diagnosed in the United States in 2005. Epidemiologists are now arguing about whether the incidence of melanoma has reached epidemic proportions or not. There have been no significant advances in the medical treatment or survival rate in the last thirty years, but if caught in the earliest stages, melanoma is treatable and has a survival rate of over 90 per cent. If untreated and allowed to spread, there is no known treatment or cure.

Whatever the outcome of present melanoma research, no one doubts that this cancer is a true health hazard and is directly attributable to sun exposure, whatever other factors might be involved. And sunlight radiation (ultraviolet A and ultraviolet B) is responsible for a host of other problems, including skin damage, wrinkles and aging-skin disorders, not to mention suppressed immunity against infection.

Ultraviolet radiation is also one of the major creators of free radicals. Through mechanisms not yet fully understood—which include impeding cell functions and damaging genetic material—the free radical cascades generated by this ionizing radiation are the agents that link radiation to disease. Through the actions of free radicals, the effects of solar radiation are nothing short of the effects of cartoon ray guns—just slower and less obvious.

How can we protect ourselves from this force of nature? First, by covering up with protective clothing. Second, by using an appropriate grade of chemical-free suntan lotion. And third, by taking antioxidants with high affinity to the skin, such as vitamins C and E and beta-carotene and the bioflavanoids. Of course, vitamin D is a big gift from the sun, but fifty or twenty minutes a day of exposure before 11 a.m. and after 2 p.m. is all we need, combined with vitamin supplementation.

Mobile-Telephone Radiation

More than four billion people worldwide are using cellphones. Considering that you live in an urbanized world, you're probably one of them. So am I. But though these findings are still being contested, a series of studies have indicated that cellphone wave emissions, called electromagnetic radiation (EMR), cause biological tissue destruction. And the tissue closest to hand when using a cellphone is brain tissue.

In 1993, the wireless technology industry in the United States chose Dr. George Carlo, a public health scientist, trained epidemiologist, lawyer and research and development director, to head its $28.5 million Wireless Technology Research (WTR) project. The project ended in 2000, but not before some disturbing results emerged. Carlo found evidence of health risk and biological damage caused by interference with cellular repair processes and attributable to cellphone radiation exposure. He found a doubling in the risk of a rare type of brain cancer among cellphone users, including a strong correlation between the site of the tumours and the side of the head where the phones were used.

The cellphone signal is called an information-carrying radio wave (ICRW). "It is completely man-made," says Dr. Carlo. Since there's nothing like it in nature, when vibration sensors on a cell membrane feel that radio wave, they interpret it as a foreign invader. "The cell membrane closes down pathways, known as active transport channels, in an effort to protect itself."

These are the same pathways that allow your trillions of cells to exchange nutrients and antioxidants. "When the ICRW is constant over a period of time," Dr. Carlo explains, "the cell membrane configures chronically in this state of sympathetic lock. When that happens, nutrients cannot enter the cell and waste products cannot leave. The cell now becomes energy deficient and intercellular communication is compromised. When cells can't talk to each other, they cannot function as tissues and organs—thus, it becomes a systemic problem."

The consequence of that systemic problem, Dr. Carlo explained to me, is a compromised immune system. With disrupted intercellular communication, the signals your cells send out to your immune cells (the macrophages and T-cells) aren't efficient, and it becomes harder for your body to fight infection. Because waste products aren't moving out of your cells, free radicals build up, attacking the mitochondria (the little energy-producing organelles inside your cells) and interfering with normal DNA repair among other things. Dr. Carlo's research points out that the resulting genetic damage can include the formation of intercellular micronuclei that under certain circumstances can clone, proliferate and lead to the development of tumours. "The other conditions that we have seen in our clinics and registries," Dr. Carlo says, "range from sleep disturbances, memory loss, focus problems and learning deficits to endocrine, nervous, digestive, reproductive and immune system compromise."

Carlo, who is now the chair of the non-profit Science and Public Policy Institute in Washington, D.C., has since conducted many scientific reviews of evidence on the effects of cellphone use, including a Danish study that found that cellphones were not harmful. As a result of his findings, he has launched the Safe Wireless Initiative, established to promote safety and empower consumers to protect themselves and their families. You can find the initiative online at www.safewireless.org, where among other things you can download intervention recommendations to help you minimize your own exposure. I also recommend the book Dr. Carlo co-wrote with Martin Schram, called *Cell Phones: Invisible Hazards in the Wireless Age,* which also describes the lack of industry response to the recommendations and findings of the original study Dr. Carlo undertook on their behalf.

Dr. Carlo believes we are on the front end of a health risk epidemic caused by the unbridled expansion of wireless communication worldwide. In the United States and Canada there are more than one million base station antennas that emit ICRW twenty-four hours a day. Carlo and his research collaborators published a paper in November 2008 (in the *Australasian Journal of Nutritional Environmental Medicine*) that was the first to link autism with electromagnetic radiation exposure. Dr. Carlo argues that for health-care practitioners to treat patients effectively they have to take into account the impact that our constant exposure to such electromagnetic radiation has on our immune systems, and the ever rising accumulation of free radicals from that ever rising tide of radiation. Since ICRW affects the transport channels of cells, antioxidants are going to have just as tough a time passing into cells as other substances and are going to be less effective as a result.

This is not good news for any of us. I can only caution you as I caution myself. We are blessed with efficient land-line telephone systems in North America. Let's significantly limit our use of cellphones.

TOXIC CHEMICALS AND SOME HELPFUL ANTIOXIDANTS

Toxic Chemical	Alternative	Organ Affected	Helpful Antioxidant
BFRs (Brominated Flame Retardants) BFRs are used to slow the spread of fire in carpets and contain PBDEs (polybrominated diphenyl ethers), a group of chemicals that are highly persistent and bioconcentrating; they are suspected hormone disruptors and can cause cancer and reproductive and developmental disorders.	Organic or natural-fibre carpets, such as wool, cotton, rattan or jute	**Thyroid and Nervous System** PBDEs are suspected of having particularly damaging effects on the thyroid (which controls brain development) and, as a result, PBDEs may cause neurodevelopmental disorders such as learning disabilities and behaviour problems. PBDEs leach from products and have been detected in house dust, human blood and breast milk.	Vitamin A
			A great way to reduce your toxic exposure in the first place is to have lots of house plants. Houseplants clean air by absorbing chemicals and converting them into food and energy. Top air cleaners include philodendron, Boston fern, peace lily and English ivy. It is recommended that homes have 2–3 houseplants per 10 m^2 (100 sq. ft.) of room space.
PVC (Polyvinyl Chloride) PVC is a harmful plastic that emits toxic chemicals (including bisphenol A polycarbonate). PVC is used to make construction materials (such as pipes, flooring and wiring) and a range of consumer products (computers, DVD and VHS players, plastic bottles and containers, baby bottles, toys, records and clothes). These plastics are labelled #3, #6 and #7. (The number is usually found on the bottom of the item inside a recycle symbol.)	Drink from glass containers, stainless steel, or plastics #1, #2, #4 and #5. Use naturally sourced flooring such as cork or rubber. Turn off your electronic devices when not in use. NOTE: Dell is phasing out brominated flame retardants and PVC by 2009, and Nokia, Samsung and Sony are following suit.	**Endocrine System** The manufacturing of PVC involves the use and emission of dioxin, but more importantly for the health of humans, PVC products can leach toxic additives, such as phthalates, throughout their use. Phthalates are added to PVC products to make them softer and more flexible, but these chemicals are known to disrupt hormones, leading to birth defects of male reproductive organs.	Indole-3-carbinol (I3C)

TOXIC CHEMICALS AND SOME HELPFUL ANTIOXIDANTS

Toxic Chemical	Alternative	Organ Affected	Helpful Antioxidant
PFOS and PFOA (Perfluorinated Chemicals) PFOS is used as a stain repellent on clothing and other fabric products such as carpets. This chemical is also used in food packaging, particularly for fast food and microwave popcorn bags. PFOA is used to make Gore-Tex and Teflon products such as non-stick cookware.	Don't worry about a little stain or a little pan stick!	**Endocrine and Immune Systems** Studies suggest that these chemicals can cause cancer and disrupt hormones.	Glutathione Ingredients to support naturally derived "superoxide dismutase": <ul><li>Zinc</li><li>Copper</li><li>Selenium</li><li>Manganese</li></ul>
OPs (Organochlorine Pesticides) There are many different types of pesticides, insecticides, fungicides and other chemical treatments used in agriculture and lawn care, and for the treatment of pests such as mosquitoes and moths. OPs are mainly used on agricultural crops—meaning on the fruits and vegetables we all eat. These chemicals are highly toxic and persistent in the environment. **Top 10 most contaminated fruits/ vegetables***: Peaches Strawberries Apples Cherries Sweet Bell Peppers Pears Celery Grapes (Imported) Nectarines Spinach	Organic pesticide-free produce	**Multiple Systems** OPs have been shown to cause cancer, skeletal abnormalities and reproductive, neurological and immune system damage.	Glutathione N-acetylcysteine Ingredients to support naturally derived "superoxide dismutase": <ul><li>Zinc</li><li>Copper</li><li>Selenium</li><li>Manganese</li></ul>

*From the Environmental Working Group

TOXIC CHEMICALS AND SOME HELPFUL ANTIOXIDANTS

Toxic Chemical	Alternative	Organ Affected	Helpful Antioxidant
PERC (Perchloroethylene) The most common form of dry cleaning uses a chemical called perchloroethylene (or PERC).	Machine-washable clothing and biodegradable detergent. For any dry-cleaning, seek out non-toxic providers.	**Nervous System** Even short-term exposure to PERC can cause adverse health effects on the nervous system. Contact with PERC in its liquid or vapour form can irritate the skin, eyes, nose and throat. Long-term exposure to PERC can cause liver and kidney damage. PERC has been shown to cause cancer in laboratory animals that repeatedly breathed PERC in air.	Alpha-lipoic acid
Phthalates Phthalates are found in cosmetics, toiletries and perfumes with synthetic fragrances.	Chemical-free products manufactured by: Aubrey Organics, Avalon, Aveda, Burt's Bees, Dr. Bronner, Druide, Ecco Bella, Jason, Kiss My Face, Mill Creek, Nature's Gate	**Reproductive System** Scientific research has shown that phthalates disrupt hormones and can cause birth defects of male reproductive organs.	Zinc Selenium
VOCs (Volatile Organic Compounds) VOCs are found in paints, varnishes, paint-stripping products, gasoline, glue, adhesives and solvents.	Products that are water based, plant-oil based and those that have low-level VOCs.	**Liver**	Glutathione

TOXIC CHEMICALS AND SOME HELPFUL ANTIOXIDANTS

Toxic Chemical	Alternative	Organ Affected	Helpful Antioxidant
HEAVY METALS **Mercury** Mercury is found in dental amalgams and tainted fish, such as tuna, and in water and air (still produced by coal-burning power plants).	Switch to composite resins in teeth. Avoid large, predatory fish such as tuna and swordfish.	**Brain and Nervous System** There are absolutely no safe levels of mercury. This heavy metal causes degeneration of nerve fibres and connectivity of neurons in the brain.	Alpha–lipoic acid
Lead Lead is found in paint, crystal glass, pipes, certain cosmetics, and hair dyes.	Paints made from natural raw ingredients such as water, plant oils and resins, plant dyes, and essential oils; natural minerals such as clay, chalk and talcum; and milk casein, natural latex, bees' wax, earth and mineral dyes. These paints are the safest for your health and for the environment.	**Immune and Nervous Systems**	Vitamin C Alpha–lipoic acid Selenium Vitamin E
Arsenic (a.k.a. CCA-pressure-treated wood) Arsenic is used for patios and fences (it has a green tint to it and leaches arsenic). Arsenic is also found in water and in high concentrations in cigarettes.	Non-CCA pressure-treated wood	**Blood Circulation, Cell Chromosome Aberrations, Kidneys and Nervous System**	N-acetylcysteine Alpha–lipoic acid

FOOD ADDITIVES

Here are some of the most common additives and preservatives and what we know about their side effects.

FOOD ADDITIVES

Acesulfame Potassium   Artificial sweetener found in baked goods,
                                           chewing gum, gelatin, desserts, soft drinks.

Manufactured by Hoechst, a giant German chemical company, and widely used around the
world. It is about 200 times sweeter than sugar. In the United States, for several years
acesulfame-K (the K is the chemical symbol for potassium) was permitted only in such
foods as sugar-free baked goods, chewing gum and gelatin desserts. In July 1998, the FDA
allowed this chemical to be used in soft drinks, thereby greatly increasing consumer exposure. Health Canada's Food Protection Branch also finds this substance to be safe.

Safety tests were conducted in the 1970s and were of mediocre quality. Disease in the
animal colonies affected key rat tests; a mouse study was several months short and did not
expose animals during gestation. Two rat studies suggested that the additive might cause
cancer. It was for those reasons that in 1996 the Center for Science in the Public Interest
urged the FDA to require better testing before permitting acesulfame-K in soft drinks. In
addition, large doses of acetoacetamide, a breakdown product, have been shown to affect
the thyroid in rats, rabbits and dogs. With luck, the small amounts in food are not harmful.

Artificial Colour Blue No. 1   In beverages, candy and baked goods. Most
                                           artificial colourings are chemicals that do
                                           not occur in nature. Because colourings are
                                           used almost solely in foods of low nutritional
                                           value, you should simply avoid all artificially
                                           coloured foods. In addition to the problems
                                           mentioned below, colour additives cause
                                           hyperactivity in some sensitive children.

Inadequately tested; suggestions of a small cancer risk.

Artificial Colour Blue No. 2   Pet food, beverages, candy.
                                           Do not ingest.

The largest study suggested, but did not prove, that this dye caused brain tumours in male
mice. The FDA concluded that there is "reasonable certainty of no harm."

Artificial Colour Green No. 3   Candy, beverages. To be avoided.

A 1981 industry-sponsored study gave hints of bladder cancer, but the FDA reanalyzed the
data using other statistical tests and concluded that the dye was safe. Fortunately, this
possibly carcinogenic dye is rarely used.

Artificial Colour Red No. 3   Cherries in fruit cocktail, candy, baked
                                           goods. Do not ingest.

The evidence that this dye caused thyroid tumours in rats is "convincing," according to a
1983 review committee report requested by the FDA. The FDA's recommendation that the
dye be banned was overruled.

FOOD ADDITIVES

Artificial Colour Yellow No. 6

Beverages, sausage, baked goods, candy, gelatin. Avoid.

Industry-sponsored animal tests indicated that this dye, the third most widely used colouring in the food industry, causes tumours of the adrenal gland and kidney. In addition, small amounts of several carcinogens contaminate Yellow No. 6. However, the FDA reviewed those data and found reasons to conclude that Yellow No. 6 does not pose a significant cancer risk to humans. Yellow No. 6 may also cause occasional allergic reactions.

Aspartame (Equal, NutraSweet)

Artificial sweetener: Diet foods, including soft drinks, drink mixes, gelatin desserts, low-calorie frozen desserts, packets.

Aspartame, a chemical combination of two amino acids and methanol, was initially thought to be the perfect artificial sweetener, but it might cause cancer or neurological problems such as dizziness or hallucinations. A 1970s study suggested that aspartame caused brain tumours in rats. However, the FDA persuaded an independent review panel to reverse its conclusion that aspartame was unsafe. The California Environmental Protection Agency and others have urged that independent scientists conduct new animal studies to resolve the cancer question. In 2005, researchers at the Ramazzini Foundation in Bologna, Italy, conducted the first such study. It indicated that some female rats first exposed to aspartame at eight weeks of age developed lymphomas and leukemias. However, the European Food Safety Authority reviewed the study and concluded that the tumours probably occurred by chance. In 2007, the same Italian researchers published a follow-up study that began exposing rats to aspartame in utero. This study found that aspartame caused leukemias/lymphomas and mammary (breast) cancer.

In a 2006 study, U.S. National Cancer Institute researchers studied a large number of adults 50 to 69 years of age exposed to aspartame over a five-year period. There was no evidence that aspartame posed any risk. However, the study was limited in three major regards: it did not involve truly elderly people (the rat studies monitored the rats until they died), the subjects had not consumed aspartame as children, and it was not a controlled study (the subjects provided only a rough estimate of their aspartame consumption, and people who consumed aspartame might have had other dietary or lifestyle differences that obscured the chemical's effects).

As far as I'm concerned I recommend that people—especially young children—do not consume foods and beverages sweetened with aspartame and either switch to products sweetened with sucralose (Splenda) or avoid all artificially sweetened foods.

Cyclamate

Banned.

This controversial high-potency sweetener was used in the United States in diet foods until 1970, at which time it was banned. Animal studies indicated that it causes cancer. Now, based on animal studies, it (or a by-product) is believed not to cause cancer directly, but to increase the potency of other carcinogens and to harm the testes. Cyclamate is also banned in Canada.

FOOD ADDITIVES

Trans-Fats: hydrogenated and partially   Fat, oil, shortening, margarine, crackers,
hydogenated vegetable oil   fried restaurant foods, baked goods.

Vegetable oil, usually a liquid, can be made into a semi-solid shortening through a reaction with hydrogen. Now facing widening bans, partial hydrogenation reduces the levels of polyunsaturated oils and also creates trans-fats, which promote heart disease. A committee of the FDA concluded in 2004 that on a gram-for-gram basis, trans-fat is even more harmful than saturated fat. Food manufacturers are moving to replace hydrogenated shortening with less-harmful ingredients. The Institute of Medicine has advised consumers to consume as little trans-fat as possible, ideally less than about 2 g a day (that much might come from naturally occurring trans-fat in beef and dairy products). Harvard School of Public Health researchers estimate that trans-fat has caused about 50,000 premature heart attack deaths annually, making partially hydrogenated oil one of the most harmful ingredients in the food supply.

Usually the substitutes being used are healthier. Foods labelled "0 g trans-fat" are permitted to contain 0.5 g per serving, whereas "no trans-fat" means none at all. Consumers need to read labels carefully: foods labelled "0 g trans" or "no trans" may still have large amounts of saturated fat.

Restaurants have been slower to change, but the pace of change is picking up. Partially hydrogenated oil is used for frying chicken, potatoes and fish, as well as in biscuits and other baked goods. Wendy's, KFC, Taco Bell, Ruby Tuesday and Red Lobster are some of the large chains that have largely eliminated trans-fat or soon will. McDonald's, the largest chain, expects to complete the changeover sometime in 2008. Most large chains and many smaller independent restaurants continue to fry food in partially hydrogenated oil, and their french fries, fried chicken, fried fish and pot pies contain substantial amounts of trans-fat.

In 2004, the Center for Science in the Public Interest (CSPI) petitioned the FDA to immediately require restaurants to disclose when they use partially hydrogenated oil and to begin the process of eliminating partially hydrogenated oil from the entire food supply. Although the FDA rejected the idea of requiring restaurants to disclose the presence of trans-fat, New York City, Philadelphia and other jurisdictions have set tight limits on the trans-fat content of restaurant foods. Meanwhile, the FDA is continuing to consider CSPI's petition to revoke the legal status of partially hydrogenated oil (the FDA considers the oil to be "generally recognized as safe," even though it and everyone else considers it to be "generally recognized as dangerous").

Fully hydrogenated vegetable oil does not have any trans-fat, but it also does not have any polyunsaturated oils. It is sometimes mixed (physically or chemically) with polyunsaturated liquid soybean oil to create trans-fat-free shortening. When it is chemically combined with liquid oil, the ingredient is called inter-esterified vegetable oil. Meanwhile, oil processors are trying to improve the hydrogenation process so that less trans-fat forms.

FOOD ADDITIVES

Olestra (Olean)   Fat substitute: in chips, crackers.

Olestra is Procter & Gamble's synthetic fat, which is not absorbed by the body, but runs right through it. Procter & Gamble suggests that replacing regular fat with Olestra will help people lose weight and lower the risk of heart disease. Olestra can cause diarrhea and loose stools, abdominal cramps, flatulence and other adverse effects. Those symptoms are sometimes severe.

Even more importantly, Olestra reduces the body's ability to absorb fat-soluble carotenoid antioxidants (such as alpha- and beta-carotene, lycopene, lutein and canthaxanthin) from fruits and vegetables. Those nutrients are thought by many experts to reduce the risk of cancer and heart disease. Olestra enables manufacturers to offer greasy-feeling low-fat snacks, but consumers would be much better off with baked snacks, which are perfectly safe and just as low in calories. Products made with Olestra should not be called "fat free," because they contain substantial amounts of indigestible fat.

Potassium Bromate   Flour improver: in bread and rolls.

This additive has long been used to increase the volume of bread and to produce bread with a fine crumb structure. Most potassium bromate rapidly breaks down to form innocuous bromide. However, potassium bromate itself causes cancer in animals. The tiny amounts of the additive that may remain in bread pose a small risk to consumers, but the substance has been banned worldwide except in Japan and the United States.

Propyl Gallate   Preservative: vegetable oil, meat products, potato sticks, chicken soup base, chewing gum. Avoid.

Propyl gallate retards the spoilage of fats and oils and is often used with BHA and BHT (see chart below), because of the synergistic effects on these preservatives. The best studies on rats and mice were peppered with suggestions (but not definitive proof) that this preservative might cause cancer.

Saccharin   Artificial sweetener: diet products, soft drinks (especially fountain drinks at restaurants), single-serving packets. Avoid.

Saccharin (Sweet'N Low) is 350 times sweeter than sugar and is used in dietetic foods or as a tabletop sugar substitute. Many studies on animals have shown that saccharin can cause cancer of the bladder. In other rodent studies, saccharin has caused cancer of the uterus, ovaries, skin, blood vessels and other organs. Other studies have shown that saccharin increases the potency of other cancer-causing chemicals. And the best epidemiology study (done by the National Cancer Institute) found that the use of artificial sweeteners (saccharin and cyclamate) was associated with a higher incidence of bladder cancer.

In 1977, the FDA proposed that saccharin be banned, because of studies that showed that it causes cancer in animals. However, Congress intervened and permitted it to be used, provided that foods bear a warning notice. It has been replaced in many products by aspartame (NutraSweet). In 1997, the diet-food industry began pressuring the U.S. and Canadian governments and the World Health Organization to take saccharin off their lists of cancer-causing chemicals. The industry acknowledges that saccharin causes bladder cancer in male rats, but argues that those tumours are caused by a mechanism that would not occur in humans. Many public-health experts respond by stating that, even if that still-unproved mechanism were correct in male rats, saccharin could cause cancer by additional mechanisms and that, in some studies, saccharin has caused bladder cancer in mice and in female rats and other cancers in both rats and mice.

In May 2000, the U.S. Department of Health and Human Services removed saccharin from its list of cancer-causing chemicals. Later that year, Congress passed a law removing the warning notice that likely will result in increased use in soft drinks and other foods and in a slightly greater incidence of cancer.

Sodium Nitrite and Sodium Nitrate

Preservative, colouring, flavouring: bacon, ham, frankfurters, luncheon meats, smoked fish, corned beef. Avoid.

Meat processors love sodium nitrite because it stabilizes the red colour in cured meat (without nitrite, hot dogs and bacon would look grey) and gives a characteristic flavour. Sodium nitrate is used in dry-cured meat because it slowly breaks down into nitrite. Adding nitrite to food can lead to the formation of small amounts of potent cancer-causing chemicals (nitrosamines), particularly in fried bacon. Nitrite, which also occurs in saliva and forms from nitrate in several vegetables, can undergo the same chemical reaction in the stomach. Companies now add ascorbic acid or erythorbic acid to bacon to inhibit nitrosamine formation, a measure that has greatly reduced the problem. Although nitrite and nitrate cause only a small risk, they are still worth avoiding.

Several studies have linked consumption of cured meat and nitrite by children, pregnant women and adults with various types of cancer. Although those studies have not yet proven that eating nitrite in bacon, sausage and ham causes cancer in humans, pregnant women would be prudent to avoid those products.

The meat industry justifies its use of nitrite and nitrate by claiming that it prevents the growth of bacteria that cause botulism poisoning. That's true, but freezing and refrigeration also do that, and the U.S. Department of Agriculture has developed a safe curing method that uses lactic acid–producing bacteria. Because nitrite is used primarily in fatty, salty foods, consumers also have important nutritional reasons for avoiding nitrite-preserved foods.

Of course, we ask more of food than that it doesn't poison us. We want it to look fresh, too, even when it isn't. We want it to smell good, feel good and taste good. The food industry continues to respond to such desires with an array of enhancers.

Here are a few additives you can chew on the next time you open a package of chips, cookies or, in fact, any processed food. Only limited literature supports the idea that these substances have negative side effects, but manufacturers know that consumers are beginning to look for them because consumers increasingly attribute side effects to them. I call them the "sneaky additives" because manufacturers use a variety of derivatives and acronyms to identify these substances, and the names are hard to keep track of. Here are a few to watch for.

THE SNEAKY ADDITIVES*
Additive

Function

BHT and BHA
(butylated hydroxytoluene and
butylated hydroxyanisole)

Also Known As . . .
BOA
- tert-butyl-4-hydroxyanisole
- (1,1-dimethylethyl)-4-methoxyphenol
- tert-butyl-4-methoxyphenol
- antioxyne B
- other various trade names

BHT is a preservative used in cereals, chewing gum, potato chips, oils, etc. Residues occur in human fat. It is considered unnecessary or is easily replaced by safe substitutes. BHA retards rancidity in fats, oils and oil-containing foods. This synthetic chemical can be replaced by safer antioxidants such as vitamin E.

Carmine

Also Known As . . .
Cochineal extract

A colouring extracted from the eggs of the cochineal beetle, which lives on cactus plants in Peru, the Canary Islands and elsewhere. The actual substance that provides the colouring is carminic acid. Used in some red, pink or purple candy, yogurt, Campari, ice cream, and many other foods and beverages. Has caused allergic reactions that range from hives to anaphylactic shock. This colouring should be banned outright or at the very least food and beverage labels should identify clearly the presence of the substance. The label should also disclose that the substance is extracted from insects so that vegetarians et al. can avoid products that contain it.

MSG (Monosodium Glutamate)

The following chemicals contain MSG:
- Autolyzed plant protein
- Autolyzed yeast
- Calcium caseinate
- Gelatin
- Glutamate
- Glutamic acid
- Hydrolyzed plant protein (HPP)
- Hydrolyzed vegetable protein (HVP)
- Monopotassium glutamate

*Adapted from Center for Science in the Public
Interest: www.cspinet.org/reports/chemcuisine.htm*

This chemical brings out the flavour in many foods. Although that may sound like a treat for taste buds, the use of MSG allows companies to reduce the amount of real ingredients in their foods, such as chicken in chicken soup. In the 1960s, it was discovered that large amounts of MSG fed to infant mice destroyed nerve cells in the brain. After that research was publicized, public pressure forced baby-food companies to stop adding MSG to their products (it was used to make the foods taste better to parents). Studies have shown that some people are sensitive to MSG. Reactions include headache, nausea, weakness and burning sensation in the back of the neck and forearms. Some people complain of wheezing, changes in heart rate and difficulty breathing.

Additive	Function

Mycoprotein

Also Known As . . .
- Sodium caseinate
- Textured protein
- Yeast extract
- Yeast food or nutrient

A novel ingredient in Quorn frozen meat substitutes, made from a processed mould (*Fusarium venenatum*). This is not a fungus or mushroom protein but a mould grown in liquid solution in large tanks. It has been used in the UK since the 1990s, and also sold in other parts of the European Union, and it has been available in North America since 2002. The fungus is nutritious, but some consumers have had allergic reactions, from vomiting to diarrhea, hives to anaphylactic shock. The incidence of sensitivity to mycoprotein is about the same as other food allergies, such as allergies to peanut, soy and milk.

Sodium benzoate, benzoic acid

A preservative in fruit juice, carbonated drinks, pickles, which manufacturers have used for at least a century to prevent the growth of microorganisms in food. The substances also occur naturally in many plants and animals. They are safe for most people, though they can cause hives, asthma and other allergic reactions in people with food sensitivities, and in some children, especially those with attention deficity hyperactivity / disorder, they may adversely affect behaviour.

Another problem comes when the substance is used in beverages that also contain vitamin C, or ascorbic acid. The two can react to produce small amounts of benzene, a chemical that causes leukemia and other cancers. In the early 1990s, the FDA urged companies not to use sodium benzoate in products that also contain ascorbic acid, but some companies still use the combination. A lawsuit filed in 2006 ultimately forced CocaCola, PepsiCo, and other soft-drink makers in the United States to reformulate affected beverages, typically fruit-flavoured products.

Sulfites

Agents that prevent discolouration in dried fruit, some "fresh" shrimp and some dried, fried or frozen potatoes. They prevent bacterial growth in wine too. They also destroy vitamin B-1. They can cause severe reactions, especially in asthmatics. Safe for individuals. Though you need to be sure you are non-sensitive as the additive caused at least twelve identifiable deaths in the 1980s. Severe reactions were most often assciated with food from restaurants, as restaurant workers would often leave lettuce or potatoes sitting in sulfite solutions. As a result of pressure from the CSPI, a

Additive	Function
Sulfites (continued)	Congressional hearing and media attention, the FDA banned the most dangerous uses of sulfites and required that wine labels list sulfites when used.
Tartrazine (Yellow No. 5) **Also Known As . . .** • FD&C Yellow No. 5 • E-102	Seeing that Yellow Nos. 1, 2, 3 and 4 are all in the "Food Additive Cemetery," it's time for Nos. 5 and 6 to follow suit.

Most people may not be able to pronounce the names of many of these chemicals, but they still want to know what the chemicals do and which ones are safe and which are poorly tested or possibly dangerous. A simple rule about additives is to avoid those found in the two charts above. Not only are they among the most questionable additives, but they are also used primarily in foods of low nutritional value.

—

USEFUL MEDICAL TESTS AND LABORATORY PROVIDERS

MEDICAL TESTS

Let's look at how you and your doctor can use the current standard blood tests to screen you for antioxidant status and free radical activity.

The type of blood work that your doctor typically and properly runs on you every year during your annual physical is called a *blood chemistry and CBC (complete blood count) evaluation.* A physical is also usually augmented by a number of other standard tests that relate to your age, gender and personal medical history. Results from such tests can be interpreted to give clues to whether or not your body is dealing well with excess free radicals or is deficient in antioxidants, and these results may suggest you need further analysis. Ask your doctor to discuss these findings with you—a single finding, like a single symptom, does not necessarily mean that there is a problem, but it often warrants a retest.

Dr. Dicken Weatherby and Dr. Scott Ferguson are the authors of seven books in the field of functional diagnosis, including *Blood Chemistry and CBC Analysis*. Both naturopathic doctors, they are actively involved in research, writing, teaching and private practice. I've based much of the content of the table below on their research.

As a testament to the quality of their work, I use their book as a primary source when tutoring an adjunctive lab analysis course to second- and third-year students at the Ontario College of Homeopathic Medicine.

All of the suggestions are for information purposes only and not to indicate a diagnosis.

WHAT ROUTINE BLOOD WORK REVEALS ABOUT YOUR ANTIOXIDANT STATUS

Name and Rationale for Test	Finding	Relationship to Antioxidant Status
Triglyceride levels (Dietary fat analysis to interpret cardiovascular health, among other things)	Abnormally low	Excess oxidative stress or free radical pathology can be the result of endurance exercise or chemical or heavy-metal overload, all of which cause triglyceride levels to plummet.
Cholesterol level (Steroid component of the immune system and cell membrane.) To analyze dietary habits, cardiovascular risk and liver status	Abnormally low* (*Unoxidized cholesterol acts as a natural antioxidant and a free radical scavenger in the body, so decreased levels put the body at risk of developing oxidative stress, and increase the chance of free radical-induced disease.)	Excess oxidative stress and free radical activity

Name and Rationale for Test	Finding	Relationship to Antioxidant Status
LDL (Dubbed the "bad" cholesterol since it is most likely to deposit on your artery walls and block blood flow)	High (It is not cholesterol in and of itself that causes blocked arteries, but rather the initial free radical injury to the artery by oxidative stress, and then the deposit of cholesterol to that injury site.)	Increased oxidative stress and free radical activity The free radical attack on LDL promotes the accumulation of plaque formation.
HDL (Dubbed the "good" cholesterol because it functions to recycle cholesterol but isn't as likely as LDL to deposit on your artery wall)	Low	Acts as an antioxidant and free radical scavenger Decreased levels means you are at greater risk of free radical damage.
LDL (Dubbed the "bad" cholesterol since it is most likely to deposit on your artery walls and block blood flow)	High (It is not cholesterol in and of itself that causes blocked arteries, but rather the initial free radical injury to the artery by oxidative stress, and then the deposit of cholesterol to that injury site.)	Increased oxidative stress and free radical activity The free radical attack on LDL promotes the accumulation of plaque formation.
Uric Acid (Assesses inflammatory or circulatory disorders such as gout, heart disease and oxidative stress)	High (or "high-normal") (Remind your doctor that if the uric acid level is increased while total cholesterol level is suddenly low, along with a decreased lymphocyte count, decreased albumin and platelet levels, and increased total globulin, there should be further investigation into free radical activity to rule out tumour.)	Oxidative stress and increased free radical activity

Name and Rationale for Test	Finding	Relationship to Antioxidant Status
Albumin (Assesses hydration levels and digestive status)	Low or steady decrease	Oxidative stress and free radical activity is high or developing, often with fluid retention (edema)
Globulin (Investigates inflammatory or immune disturbances as well as digestive status)	Increased	Excess oxidative stress and free radical activity
ALT/AST/ALP/GGT (Liver enzymes representative of overall detoxification status)	Increased (any one or all)	Reduced toxin clearance capacity causing free radicals to accumulate
Total Bilirubin (Monitors red blood cell breakdown and/or blockage of bile in the liver)	High	Oxidative stress can cause an increased destruction in red blood cells, of which increased levels of bilirubin is a sign.
White Blood Count (Monitors the body's ability to respond to infection)	Elevated	Possible free radical pathology (i.e., infection or tumour)
Lymphocyte (Screens body's defence system)	Decreased or Low	Oxidative stress and free radical activity
Reticulocyte Count (Rules out chronic internal [invisible] bleeding and diagnoses proper form of anemia)	Increased	Free radical pathology Deficient vitamin C Heavy metal toxicity Liver dysfunction
Platelet (Evaluates bleeding disorder)	Low	Oxidative stress and free radical activity

Testing Part Two

You can assay your approximate antioxidant demands with the antioxidant calculator in this book, test at home with my antioxidant test kit, and ask your doctor for further annual screening. The following are even more tests you may wish to undergo in order to get a full free radical work-up. At the molecular level, as we saw, free radicals are at the root of every known disease. But because free radicals are part of our immune system's arsenal in its defence against harmful infectious viruses and bacteria, the testing of optimal individual levels can be tricky. The determination of an *imbalance* between the production of free radicals and the ability of our natural protective mechanisms to cope with them is the critical objective. Just as in the case of our blood cholesterol levels, a reading that is too high is dangerous, but having too low a reading can be a problem too. To get the most accurate picture, both blood and urine can be tested to determine antioxidant status and free radical levels. And since numerous studies suggest that lipids (fats), proteins and DNA are the cellular components that are most sensitive to damage induced by free radicals, when we attempt to assess antioxidant status, we measure the degree of free radical damage on lipids, proteins and DNA.

If I get a teeny bit technical in this section, it's because it's important to know exactly what these tests are and what they represent in order to ask your health-care provider to run them for you. The quantities of these biomarkers represent the degree of free radical damage to the cells. The findings of a higher than normal value indicates free radical damage, and therefore an increased demand for various antioxidants.

Finding Damage to Your Cell Membrane

Human cell membranes (the external shell) contain polyunsaturated fatty acids (PUFAs), which are among the most oxygen-sensitive molecules in nature. Certain properties of PUFAs act in a cell-signalling capacity. They do not require a prior activation of genes, but are the by-product of a non-specific response to a variety of external or internal health impacts. When due to, say, the attack of a micro-organism or a change in temperature, the amount of liberated free PUFAs exceeds a certain threshold and the cells commit suicide.

There is very strong evidence from animal studies that another biomarker called 8-epi-prostaglandin PGF2a (8-epi-PGF2a) increases in plasma and urine as a result of oxidative and free radical stress. A number of investigators have suggested that it may be a reliable test of free radical generation and oxidative lipid formation. When smokers are tested, 8-epi-PGF2a is always present at elevated levels. Its formation is modulated by antioxidant status, and its level is not affected by the fat content of a diet. As long as antioxidants such as glutathione and vitamin C are available, the amount of damage is kept low.

Protein Oxidation: Discovering Damage to Your Body's Tissues and Organs

Free radical damage can affect proteins and give rise to molecules called protein *carbonyl derivatives*. This protein oxidation has a lethal effect on the normal functioning of our bodies, since every tissue, including our connective tissue (skin, cartilage, blood vessels, etc.), is made of protein. Much of the consequence of visible aging—aging of the skin, for example—correlates to this biomarker. There are two chemicals in the body—2-oxohistine and nitrotyrosine—that are thought to be an indicator of protein damage induced by free radicals. You can test for free radical damage to your body protein by testing a blood sample for these markers. The antioxidants of choice for good results are the water-soluble nutrients: vitamin C, alpha-lipoic acid and bioflavanoids. It is a little-known fact that many of the supplemental amino acids act in ways that are both reparative to your body protein and also act as an antioxidant to neutralize free radical damage that causes disease and aging.

G6PD: A Battle between Red Blood Cells and Free Radicals

G6PD deficiency is a hereditary abnormality in the activity of a red blood cell enzyme and is the most common enzyme deficiency in the world. This enzyme, glucose-6-phosphate dehydrogenase (G6PD), is essential for assuring a normal lifespan for red blood cells, and for oxidizing processes. The enzyme deficiency may provoke the sudden destruction of red blood cells; if you have this abnormality, a deadly type of anemia may be triggered by eating fava beans, certain legumes or taking various drugs such as antimalarial and anti-itching medications.

Because G6PD is carried on the X chromosome, the defect is transmitted from the mother (usually healthy herself and simply a carrier) to her son (or daughter, who would be a healthy carrier too). Males have an XY chromosome and are at risk of whatever gender-linked diseases may come from the mother (the only provider of the X chromosome). The deficit is most prevalent in Africa (affecting up to 20 per cent of the population), but it is also common around the Mediterranean and in Southeast Asia. There are more than four hundred genetic variants known. You can determine whether you are G6PD-deficient by a simple blood test that measures the actual activity of the G6PD enzyme in the blood. Because the enzyme is in charge of producing energy from sugar and helps protect cells from the damaging effects of free radicals, if there is insufficient G6PD activity inside red blood cells, these cells are more vulnerable to oxidative damage. If they are exposed to free radical molecules, their cellular structure may undergo change that affects their hemoglobin (oxygen-carrying capacity) and leads to their destruction.

Antioxidants can alleviate some of the harmful effects of free radical damage in cases of genetic diseases such as G6PD deficiency. A report in the *Journal of Biomedical Sciences* from the School of Medical Technology in Taiwan is but one study that demonstrates the effects of free radical damage on the G6PD component of human cells. As a consequence of this enhanced susceptibility to oxidative stress, G6PD-deficient individuals have lower antioxidant levels—lower vitamin C levels particularly—than normal individuals. Taking high amounts of vitamin C (1,000 mg three times daily) and glutathione (1,000 mg three times daily) may be helpful in these cases.

This condition and its treatment is more proof that you can't assume an average requirement of antioxidant supplementation for any general population. Each person possesses a unique set of genes and requires individual amounts to keep optimal. The Taiwan study also found that the red blood cell damage could be affected by two environmental pollutants: the heavy metals platinum and palladium, which can enhance the radical formation of the hydroxyl molecule in the presence of hydrogen peroxide and ferrous ion. This is called a Fenton reaction and is one of the most powerful oxidizing reactions known.

Results of a study done in Italy show that the sleep hormone melatonin (well known for its positive effects on sleep and jet lag) can act as an antioxidant that protects human red blood cells from damage. The study suggests that melatonin—just like G6PD—is actively taken up by red blood cells when under free radical attack. In our bloodstream it is the red blood cells that are constantly exposed to oxygen, and even if we don't have this disease, they can be a site for free radical formation.

DNA Destruction: Determining Damage to Your Genetic Code
One of the major products of free radical attack is—don't try to say this—8-hydroxydeoxyguanosine (8-OHdG). Numerous peer-reviewed papers have reported that there is an age-dependent increase in the level of this marker in human brain tissue. As you might suspect, people with Alzheimer's disease, Parkinson's disease and senile dementia all test at higher levels for this free radical marker.

It has been calculated that about 2 per cent of the oxygen inhaled by your lungs turns into harmful active oxygen radicals in your body. It never fails to amaze me how oxygen is our life-sustaining best friend, and in many cases also our disease-causing worst enemy. We have always to bear in mind that active oxygen is created purposely when immune cells confront invading viruses and bacteria. A small amount of free radical oxygen is essential ammunition for our bodies' immune system. However, your health is at stake when levels of this free radical type of active oxygen are dispersed in high, uncontrolled concentrations. Depending on where you live and the pollution levels in your environment, as much as 10 per cent of atmospheric oxygen can become free radical-causing oxygen in your lungs.

Deoxyguanosine is a crucial part of every strand of our DNA and a crucial ingredient of our genetic code. When it is damaged by free radicals, it is transformed into the 8-OHdG discussed above. Because free radical damage causes an oxidized state of DNA, *antioxidants* are required to neutralize that damage so that further harm is limited. Our genetic code replicates without flaw or mutation when antioxidant systems composed of enzymes, trace elements and vitamins are working to protect your genes from the onslaught of free radicals. Thankfully, we can test for the level of 8-OHdG in your blood and urine.

When DNA damage has been done, the resulting product is easily testable because it is stable in your body after it is thrown out of the affected cells and released into blood and excreted via urine. The test can measure the concentration of your 8-OHdG to determine the total free radical damage in your body, which helps your physician to evaluate your stress level, lifestyle, diet and environmental ramifications to your health.

Dr. H. Ochi, the director of the Japan Institute for the Control of Aging, has developed a refinement of the 8-OHdG test in collaboration with Professor T. Osawa at Nagoya University. A sample of blood or urine is taken and introduced into a reaction with a type of antibody that indicates only the 8-OHdG in the sample. A machine then detects the concentration of the reaction products. High readings indicate a free radical excess in the body. Specific antioxidants are required for effective treatment and prevention of disease.

Laboratories that offer this test specify that it is not intended for diagnosis but for study purposes only—the test has not yet been granted formal approval by various authorities. To be approved by these bodies, the test must offer some kind of diagnostic outcome. But there can be no diagnostic outcome because there is no "free radical disease" label because *all* disease involves free radicals.

Traditional testing is concerned with pathology. When your antioxidant status is found to be deficient or when your free radical levels are found to be high, a doctor cannot tell you, based on that, that you have any particular condition. That's why, when doctors are asked to run this test or other tests I have described, they may be sceptical of their validity, or, if they accept that the results have meaning, may not be able to present a treatment solution to you. Be prepared for this reaction. Suggest to your physician that you aren't looking for a diagnosis, but rather to understand how you may better balance free radical activity in your body by using antioxidants responsibly. He or she will probably be happy to hear you use the word "responsible" and may well send your blood or urine away for evaluation.

If enough patients pursue this course, the health-care systems in Canada and private insurance companies in the United States may begin to cover the costs of the various antioxidant-status tests sooner rather than later.

Be aware that, as with cholesterol, you will need to repeat such testing on a regular basis. I would recommend you check every three to six months in order to monitor how your status shifts through your various diets, stressful times and lifestyle changes. Once you have had perhaps four to six tests done, you'll have a reasonably good understanding of what affects your levels. Plot the results on a graph and keep a journal to record what, if any, changes happen along the way. Correlate it all to your exercise routine, supplement protocol, diet and lifestyle. Work with your holistic health-care provider to develop any insights that will help you maintain yourself at ideal levels.

LABORATORY PROVIDERS

A doctor may also resist running these incredibly important tests because he or she may not know where to send your samples. There are quality laboratories that provide the tests mentioned here. Your physician can confidently send your samples to any of the following labs for antioxidant status and other functional lab parameters.

Genova Diagnostics
63 Zillicoa St.
Asheville, NC 28801
USA
1-800-522-4762
www.gdx.net

Immunosciences Lab., Inc.
8693 Wilshire Blvd.
Beverly Hills, CA 90211
1-800-950-4686
www.immuno-sci-lab.com

Neurosciences Lab
373 280th St.
Osceola, WI 54020
USA
www.neurorelief.com

Brunswick Laboratories
50 Commerce Way
Norton, MA 02766
508-285-2006
USA
www.brunswicklabs.com

Cedarlane Laboratories Ltd.
4410 Paletta Court
Burlington, ON
Canada
L7L 5R2
(Providing high-quality
reagents to researchers and
testing facilities)
1-800-268-5058
www.cedarlanelabs.com

Northwest Lifescience
Specialties
16420 S.E. McGillvray
Suite 103, PMB 106
Vancouver, WA 98683
1-888-449-3091
www.nwlifescience.com

Doctors Data
3755 Illinois Ave.
St. Charles, IL 60174-2420
USA
1-800-323-2784
www.doctorsdata.com

Metametrix Clinical Laboratory
3425 Corporate Way
Duluth, GA 30096
USA
1-800-221-4640
www.metametrix.com

SpectraCell Laboratories
10401 Town Park Dr.
Houston, TX 77072
USA
1-800-227-5227
www.spectracell.com

The Great Plains Laboratory
11813 W 77th St.
Lenexa, KS 66214
USA
1-800-288-0383

THE TOP TEN ANTIOXIDANT QUESTIONS

You know by now what a complex subject this is and you know that solutions to health problems require a deft, holistic approach that includes good nutrition, mental and emotional balance, optimal exercise and proper oversight by qualified health-care practitioners. Nonetheless, knowledge is a valuable ally. That's why I wrote this book and that's why I offer these answers to the ten questions I am asked most frequently in my office, on my television show and during media interviews and personal appearances.

1. I want to lose weight and keep it off, but I also want to stay healthy. What pill should I take?

There is no pill that can do this job. But, if I were challenged to recommend the antioxidant pill that would make the biggest impact on weight loss—when taken in conjunction with an appropriate antioxidant nutritional plan and proper exercise it would be conjugated linoleic acid (CLA). Research suggests that CLA may help to reduce body fat and increase muscle *even without diet and exercise*. There are at least seven human studies (two are double-blind and the others are controlled ones) showing significant reduction of abdominal obesity and body fat mass in overweight and moderately obese people. I often recommend 2,000 mg of CLA three times daily.

2. How do I know that I'm getting my daily vitamin, mineral and antioxidant requirements from a "multi" or a "one-a-day"?

Other than relying on good studies that promote what may be right for the *average* person and the prevention of serious deficiencies, you *don't* know—unless you get tested. There are many tests available to screen you for specific vitamin or mineral status. However, the reason you take vitamins and minerals is to deal with the body's exposure to free radicals. So have your free radical levels tested. The Bryce Wylde Antioxidant Test Kit will give you a good indication of the control you are maintaining on your free radical burden. I recommend retesting every thirty to sixty days to ensure that you are on the right track with your diet, exercise and supplement plan. Once you've reached free radical levels that are optimal for you, you can retest every three to six months.

3. What can I take to help me sleep better at night?

Double-blind research has shown that the antioxidant melatonin facilitates sleep. It helps shorten the time it takes to get to sleep, reduces the number of night awakenings and improves sleep quality. Melatonin is also helpful in relieving symptoms of jet lag because it is also a hormone that regulates the human biological clock. Some interesting studies point towards its usefulness in treating many different types of cancer. As it is seen to play a role in regulating immunity, it is showing promise integrated into the treatment of prostate cancer, breast cancer, melanoma and some forms of brain and lung cancers. Its anti-inflammatory and strong antioxidant qualities are responsible for its anticancer properties. My recommendation as a sleep aid is often 1 mg for every 9 kg (20 lb.) of body weight, 1 hour before bed for no longer than 3 months at a time.

4. What is the single most important healthy-heart antioxidant?

Hands down, coenzyme Q_{10} (CoQ_{10}—also known as ubiquinone). The name ubiquinone describes its widespread distribution in the human body; it's found in nearly every cell and in especially high concentrations in the heart muscle tissue. CoQ_{10} is used by the body to transform food into the energy (called ATP) on which the body runs. It is a powerful antioxidant that has been shown to reduce high cholesterol, lower high blood pressure, improve symptoms of congestive heart failure and balance arrhythmias. CoQ_{10} protects the body from free radicals and helps preserve vitamin E, the major antioxidant of cell membranes and blood cholesterol. I often recommend 100 mg twice per day in a liquid gel-cap form.

5. What is the single most impressive antioxidant that you know and use yourself?

No question about this one. The answer is alpha-lipoic acid (ALA), and it's got a *long* list of uses. ALA is one of the most impressive antioxidants to surface since the discovery of vitamin C. It has been reclassified from vitamin to coenzyme antioxidant because we now know it's produced in small amounts by your body. I prescribe alpha-lipoic acid, orally, in cases of type 1 and type 2 diabetes, peripheral neuropathy, cardiac autonomic neuropathy, retinopathy, cataracts and glaucoma, dementia, chronic fatigue syndrome, HIV/AIDS, cancer, liver disease, Wilson's disease, cardiovascular disease, Lyme disease and lactic acidosis caused by inborn errors of metabolism. Intravenously, alpha-lipoic acid is used to improve insulin resistance and glucose disposal in type 2 diabetes, diabetic neuropathy and in cases of *Amanita* mushroom poisoning. This is the list of "proven" uses—even more uses are attributed to it. I often recommend a 200-mg "R+" slow-release form of ALA twice daily as part of a supplement routine.

6. Should I take antioxidants while having chemotherapy and radiation treatment?

The quick answer is no, don't take antioxidants while on a chemo/radiation protocol. Although some antioxidants may offer protection against the side effects from radiation treatment, certain antioxidants are suspected of counteracting the desired effects of chemotherapy.

But a properly educated health-care practitioner who knows your chemotherapy drugs and, more importantly, *when* you are scheduled to have them or radiation treatment can put a supportive protocol of antioxidants and perhaps other natural medicines in place. Supplementing with antioxidants at key times—such as before your chemotherapy—is the advantage that integrating conventional and natural modalities offers. Frequent testing for free radical status before, during and after treatment is advantageous to a successful outcome.

7. Can vitamins, minerals and antioxidants be harmful to your health?

Yes. Although there are no expected risks in following the personal antioxidant plan I've outlined (supplement dosages are within safe optimal daily ranges), too much of a good thing can actually do harm. Before going on a course of supplements, you must be aware of the optimal doses versus the toxic doses of the fat-soluble vitamins A, D, E and K. They can quickly accumulate to dangerous levels in the body if taken in too high doses for too long. Furthermore, when your immune system is "out of ammunition"—and your free radical levels are too *low*—you wouldn't want to supplement with high-dose antioxidants until you'd "rebooted" your immune function. Again, testing would help you to understand your current status before embarking on a daily antioxidant supplement routine.

8. What can I use to naturally help with erectile dysfunction?

L-Arginine is an amino acid that provides great cardiovascular support—most men suffering from erectile dysfunction have cardiovascular problems too. But the therapeutic ranges of L-arginine required to improve erectile dysfunction have the potential to increase nitric oxide (NO-) to harmful levels. Nitric oxide is produced in the inner lining of the blood vessels and causes the vessels to relax, allowing more blood to flow to vital body tissues and organs. But too much active nitric oxide, released too quickly, causes free radical accumulation.

So supplemental L-arginine needs to be *slowly* absorbed and metabolized by the system. Recently some excellent formulas have come onto the market that release the L-arginine into the system over a twelve-hour period. Inquire about these formulas.

9. What antioxidant is the most effective at lowering my stress levels?

There are many types of stress, including emotional stress, toxic stress and even exercise-induced stress, and there's no one supplement that fixes them all. However, there is a great deal of research to show that the antioxidant actions of the B vitamin family have powerful effects in mitigating emotional stress, improving mood, reducing homocysteine (which causes free radical attack on your arteries), lowering blood pressure and supporting nervous system function, among other things. I usually recommend 50 to 100 mg B-complex vitamin twice daily with food.

10. What antioxidant is most effective in preventing cancer?

Cancers vary enormously in how they manifest and behave, and what they require for effective treatment. What we know is that free radicals have a crucial role to play in forming cancer, and antioxidants have a crucial role to play in preventing and reversing cancers. There is no single antioxidant proven to prevent or treat all forms of cancer. Again, a single magic pill just doesn't exist. Antioxidants always work in teams. The literature overwhelmingly supports maintaining a good daily conglomerate of dozens of antioxidants to prevent cancer and protect your DNA from free radical onslaught. This is a perfect example of why I created both the antioxidant calculator in Chapter 10 as well as the test kit. If you want to prevent cancer, you'll want to know what levels of antioxidants best fit your needs. Besides the well-studied antioxidant combination ACES, here are a few that have recently caught my attention, either because they are unfamiliar antioxidants or they have had some updated and promising research:

- AHCC (active hexose-correlated compound): 500 mg once daily for prevention
- Vitamin D_3: 2,000 IU once daily for prevention
- Folic acid (5-MTF form): 800 mcg once daily for prevention
- OPCs (oligomeric proanthocyanidins): 100 mg once daily for prevention
- Glutathione (in reduced form): 500 mg twice daily for prevention
- MCP (modified citrus pectin): 15 g twice daily
- EGCG (found in green tea extract): 500 mg twice daily (containing 97% tea polyphenols and including 65% catechins) or 2 to 3 cups of green tea daily

—

CASE HISTORIES

TOXINS: HEAVY METAL-INDUCED CHRONIC FATIGUE SYNDROME OR WAS IT FIBROMYALGIA?

M. F., a thirty-eight-year-old female, presented with symptoms typical of both chronic fatigue and fibromyalgia, including debilitating fatigue and persistent muscle pain. Her antibodies tested negative for mononucleosis (the Epstein Barr virus). Testing for free radical levels showed 5 out of 5 on the urine screen and her blood serum sensitivity 8-OHdG levels were high compared to experimental models. Standard testing indicated her blood chemistry and biochemistry were otherwise unremarkable. She was approximately 30 pounds overweight, but this could not be seriously considered to be anything more than a contributing factor to her condition. Investigation for heavy metals and other toxins revealed mercury levels in a hair sample to be extremely high. A urine test also indicated the presence of mercury. Blood-borne antibodies to mercury showed significant elevation, proving *exposure* to mercury, though not the extent of the exposure.

The patient was started on a high dose of alpha-lipoic acid (300 mg) three times daily for 12 weeks as a strong antioxidant, immune regulator and mercury expeller. Doses were brought up or down over the course of treatment depending on her urine analysis results. Chelation therapy using oral Bio-Chelat was initiated for the three-month period as well.

At six months, blood work showed this patient's antibodies to mercury remained elevated, as would be expected after long exposure to the toxic metal. Free radical levels had dropped to normal ranges and heavy metals levels in her hair and urine were almost nil.

The patient reported that she was pain-free, and that her energy level was higher than it had been in ten years.

THRESHOLD: ANXIETY, THE ULTIMATE MIND-BODY DISCONNECT

K.F. is a television news anchor and respected media personality in his early forties, who seemed to develop a generalized anxiety disorder out of the blue. When I first assessed him, these episodes were bad and getting worse by the week. K.F. had been on air for years: performance anxiety wasn't the problem. His history revealed that he was not the most health-conscious eater, that he wasn't exercising, and that he was going to bed at 10 p.m. only to wake up at 2 a.m. in order to be at work by 5 a.m. He'd been following this routine for years. After running a set of adrenal competency tests and urinary MDA (to check free radical levels), it was clear that his adrenal glands were in overdrive (they control the fight-or-flight stress response).

My diagnosis was simple: a surpassed health threshold. There were multiple contributing factors. I prescribed a customized set of six different antioxidants. It took three weeks for K.F.'s free radical load to return to healthy levels. We continue to work on adrenal recuperation, breathing and relaxation techniques, an optimal diet and exercise. The good news is that he's had far fewer episodes of anxiety since starting treatment. He's still working on reducing his level of anxiety and ultimately hoping for a full remission, but without antioxidant protection he could possibly have developed heart disease and potentially lost his job.

FREE RADICALS: LUPUS A CASE OF FREE RADICAL SOUP

A. B., a thirty-six-year-old female, came to me with a diagnosis of systemic lupus erythematosus (SLE), an autoimmune condition involving the connective tissue and organs. She presented with inflammation of her joints, various skin afflictions, and blood and kidney imbalances. She also suffered from another autoimmune condition, known as Raynaud's phenomenon, which affected her circulation and made it hard for blood to reach her hands and feet. Her medical history revealed that about three years before she came to see me, she had been taking penicillin every three months for a peroid of nearly eighteen months due to repeated upper respiratory infections. These kept recurring while she was trying to work full time and go to night school. She was stressed to the max, hopping from one walk-in medical clinic to another and was never properly assessed by a family doctor. Furthermore, she was trying to get pregnant. So she was taking a whack of various synthetic hormones to try to aid her with what appeared to be infertility.

Knowing that free radicals play a major role in autoimmune and rheumatic disease, I immediately ran a battery of urine and blood tests to assess, among other things, her free radical status. All of her free radical results were through the roof: urine colormetric was 5 of 5, 8-OHdG was significantly high compared to experimental models, and her TH1/TH2 panel of cytokines (inflammatory markers) showed a major elevation of IL2 and IL10. These findings didn't represent two or more different diagnoses: This was a case of free radical soup. A. B. was swimming in inflammation.

Treatment involved specific doses of DHEA (while monitoring blood levels), R+ALA, ACES, and Kaprex—all with strong antioxidant qualities. I also put her on immune modulators, 200 mg plant sterols and sterolins three times daily, and lastly a high potency fish oil (Nutrasea HP); the dosage was 1 tsp three times daily.

A lot of stuff. But within a year, she reported that her joint pain was 60 per cent improved and that the Raynaud's phenomenon was all but gone (showing up only on the coldest winter days). She was able to maintain low free radical scores, though they crept up when she was under stress to just above normal. Though she had stopped taking the hormones (which were undoubtedly making her lupus worse), her menstrual cycles became regular. The best news of all was that she got pregnant. Furthermore, she actually showed an improvement during her pregnancy. A. B. continues to do *extremely* well.

GENETICS: DRUG SENSITIVITY, G6PD DEFICIENCY, AND AOX REPAIR

A. H. is a pleasant, slightly overweight sixty-five-year-old woman. She came to me because she had suffered from heart palpitations for more than six months. She had a pulse of 120 BPM and a very erratic heartbeat. Whenever her heart raced, she began to have anxiety attacks. In the last few months, this had become a self-perpetuating situation: getting nervous seemed to bring on the palpitations, and the palpitations, in turn, brought on nervousness.

A. H. had tried numerous drugs, but was hypersensitive to them. She was more sensitive than most people because of an inherited condition called G6PD deficiency in which the body doesn't have enough of the enzyme glucose-6-phosphate dehydrogenase to help red blood cells function normally. It is an antioxidant enzyme. Since drugs weren't going to work very well for her, I suggested a standard natural approach to try to improve her condition before her doctors next attempted a *cardioversion* (an intervention that involves resetting a patient's heart rhythm with an electrical current). I recommended that A. H. take magnesium, vitamin B6, and a high dose of liquid CoQ_{10}. This improved her symptoms slightly, but not to the degree we were looking for. Although they are often senstive to drugs, individuals with G6PD often respond well to antioxidants. (Incidentally so do people with arrhythmias.) Furthermore her blood free radicals (8-OHdG levels) were significantly high compared to experimental models.

In her circumstance, I had to be careful with the antioxidants because too high a dose of vitamin C, for example, can cause hemolytic anemia in these patients. By adding alpha-lipoic acid to her regimen, supporting her liver by adding the antioxidant glutathione, and also recommending a small antioxidant amount of melatonin, we brought her free radical levels down in short order. Once they were normalized, so too were her palpitations. The reduction in oxidative stress reduced strain on the heart muscles (and improved oxygenation). We weren't able to alter A.H.'s genes, which encoded the G6PD deficiency, but it seems that we were able to assist in controlling the expression of those genes using antioxidants to minimize the free radical burden.

AGING: A CASE OF ALZHEIMER'S DISEASE AND ARTHRITIS RESPONSIVE TO ANTIOXIDANT SYNERGY

J. W., a man in his late seventies, approached me with rheumatologic complaints. He came to my office with his distraught wife, who no longer knew what to do with him, as he was also suffering from Alzheimer's. I decided to do my best to treat the arthritis and to address, if possible, his Alzheimer's symptoms, which included bouts of depression. Without question, Alzheimer's disease is incurable once it progresses beyond a certain point. J. W. 's mental state was getting worse by the month: he would continually remind his wife of how much pain he had in his knees, hips and lower back. This was just about the only thing he didn't forget.

I didn't conduct any lab work on him because it was clear from his presentation, diagnosis and current symptoms that he would have a favourable response to antioxidant supplementation. I just didn't expect *as* good a response.

I started J. W. on a regimen of B_6, B_{12}, folic acid and SAM-e . SAM-e is a powerful antioxidant known to be effective in Alzheimer's by not only reducing free radical levels but also by increasing dopamine levels in the brain. He reported back to my office two months later and then six months after that. At the latter appointment, he and his wife reported that not only was he nearly pain free, he was much more himself: he was sleeping better, his memory was significantly improved and he was having far fewer episodes of depression.

DESTINY: GENOMIC INVESTIGATION INTO THE FUTURE OF A POPULAR TV HOST

T. R. is a thirty-two-year-old woman who competes in running and cycling races and who weight-trains. She is a very fit person who also hosts a hit TV show on fitness. She came to me for help in *maintaining* her health. I tested her DNA for possible mutations. What we found was very interesting. T. R. is in *great* shape. She works out daily, eats well, meditates, takes her antioxidants and understands what a good attitude is. Thank goodness, because if she didn't, she'd be in trouble. Her DNA revealed less than ideal variations in the genes that modulate bone formation (collagen synthesis), bone breakdown (resorption), and inflammation, including key regulatory mechanisms affecting calcium and vitamin D_3 metabolism. A problem with a gene called a VDR (vitamin D regulator) was especially troubling since it mediates the actions of vitamin D_3. Mutations in VDR can inhibit calcium absorption and decrease bone mineralization.

That meant that T. R. cannot effectively metabolize vitamin D, which is a powerful cancer- and free-radical-fighting vitamin. Her family history revealed both osteoporosis and thyroid problems. Both are vitamin D-related issues.

A mutation of the VDR gene is often mitigated by lifestyle—by remaining active and taking extra vitamin D. T. R. was doing both these things already, but after learning about this flawed gene, she stepped up her efforts.

MIND: A COMMON CASE OF DEPRESSION?

F. G., a man in his mid-fifties, came to me for help with depression. He had seen a number of other specialists for years to no avail. No one could quite get a handle on his diagnosis. It seemed like "classic" depression, but experimenting with the entire family of anti-depressants hadn't yielded any improvement and psychological counseling hadn't seemed to help him.

Free radical status testing with a simple in-house urine screening revealed a higher than acceptable range of colorimetric MDA (3 out of 5). Since F. G.'s medical history revealed no psychiatric problems other than depression, I decided to initiate treatment with some antioxidants known to be helpful in treating depression. F. G. was given optimal range vitamins A, C, E and D, along with a high-dose of folic acid and sublingual liquid B_{12}. To ensure that he was fully equipped with the necessary "brain juice" I also recommended a high dose of fish oils (10 mL twice daily). This oral therapy is typically successful because the antioxidants will cross the blood brain barrier and protect the nervous system from free radicals.

For some reason, no matter what amount of antioxidants I prescribed for F. G. during the months to come, his free radical tests always revealed an elevated 3 of 5. I was stumped. When we did more extensive blood work, we found that his serotonin levels were very low and his antibodies for serotonin were high. (The presence of such antibodies indicates that there is or was an attack by the body on its own serotonin supply.)

F. G.'s body, it seemed, was using free radicals to attack his own feel-good molecules. No wonder he felt depressed.

Adding an appropriate regime of antioxidants to neutralize this attack hadn't quite done the job because they weren't the ideal ones for the task, and his immune system was making things difficult.

To the above treatment I added a high dose of vinpocetine herb, theanine amino acid and zinc citrate. Within three to four months of beginning this customized antioxidant/immune-modulating regime, F. G. was doing much better and reported a 50 per cent improvement in his mood. Next I suggested he implement a functional meditation routine, which worked for him where no other psychological intervention had helped.

After a year in treatment, F. G. regained control over his life and reported an overall 90 per cent improvement in depression. He has since gone on to teach "lunch and learns" about mood and its health impacts at his workplace.

TESTING: TESTING FOR FREE RADICAL STATUS REVEALS CANCER

G. H. came to me in his early sixties to get help with his prostate enlargement, which was causing frequent urination, incontinence, and a "shy stream" (hesitancy). He was opposed to using any conventional medication to improve his stream, so I said that

I would be happy to recommend the indicated homeopathic medicine and a set of antioxidants indicated for his condition. His doctor had done the appropriate examination and had been tracking his PSA levels on blood work. Although slightly elevated, the levels were not increasing much over the short term.

Oxidative stress in non-metastatic prostate cancer and prostate enlargement has been well-established, so I did a free radical status panel on G. H. and found his free radical levels to be extremely elevated across the board. I prescribed the indicated antioxidants: zinc, lycopene and selenium as well as saw palmetto berry extract and the homeopathic remedy lycopodium. We rechecked his free radical levels three months later, and to my surprise they were still extremely high. I suggested we retest his PSA levels. His PSA had jumped from 5.7 nanograms per decilitre (ng/dl) to over 10 ng/dl. I put him on a high dose of inositol hexaphosphate (IP-6)—a potent antioxidant that aids in the treatment of prostate cancer—and just in case sent him back to see his doctor. An ultrasound and needle biopsy confirmed an isolated, non-metastatic prostate cancer.

Luckily a cryotherapy (freezing) application to the tumour was considered sufficient treatment. We continued the antioxidant plan with IP-6, rechecked both his PSA and his free radical status sixty days later and found that both were in normal ranges.

4 RS: RESTORING THE GUT-IMMUNE SYSTEM AND GETTING RID OF ACNE

C. S., a sixteen-year-old male, had been dealing for years with cystic acne and came to me as last resort. He had tried every application known to regular medicine and over the last year had been put on Accutane. It had not worked and had instead given him a lot of digestive trouble. A "bowel permeability" test revealed what is known in the natural health-care industry as "leaky gut syndrome." This wasn't a case for antioxidants. This was a case of dysbiosis (gut bacteria imbalance) and an irritation of the intestinal mucosal membrane. His gut-associated lymphoid tissue, which accounts for over 60 per cent of the immune system, was significantly disturbed. The need for probiotics (friendly bacteria), fish oils and L-glutamine was obvious.

I recommended these three supplements in combination with a significant overhaul in C. S.'s diet— which until then was basically pizza, chocolate milk and candy bars. Six months later his digestive system had significantly improved. He no longer had the irritable bowel that had developed after the Accutane, and his acne had cleared up by over 80 per cent. Incidentally he missed 90 per cent less school due to sickness the next year compared to the year prior.

DETOXIFICATION: FROM INFERTILE TO THE BIRTH OF A BABY IN ROUGHLY A YEAR

N. T., S. O., F. B., K. L. and B. R. were all women between the ages of thirty-one and forty-two who came to me with the same concern—infertility. Their cases (along with many others in my practice) were all identical in that they had all been trying to conceive for over two years and had been unsuccessful. After taking the usual comprehensive histories for each of them, there didn't seem to be anything obvious that was a problem. In most cases these women had tried months of monitoring their monthly cycles, hormonal treatment, IVF, or combinations of them all. (Their husbands had been ruled out as the problem. Nonetheless, I recommended that their husbands go through the same protocol that I charged them with, along with the addition of L-arginine at 1,000 mg twice daily.)

Before spending a ton of money on expensive toxicity testing, hormonal testing and investigation into any other underlying cause of their fertility, I recommended that each couple undergo a one-month "detoxification" routine involving a significant nutritional alteration and a therapeutic supplement plan, including UltraClear medical food. I've found that such a program will often push the "reset button" in the body, clearing any toxic free radical burden the person is carrying, and a successful pregnancy results. The female body seems to have an internal thermostat for impurities, and if it is registering too high, the "permission slip" for pregnancy won't easily be granted to the uterus. In each of these cases (and there are currently more than twelve of these a year in my practice), there was a successful conception and full-term pregnancy within three to seven months.

NUTRITION: A FIFTY-POUND WEIGHT LOSS IN FOUR MONTHS BY FOCUSING ON ORAC FOODS

J. L. is an extremely busy lawyer with no time to exercise: when he came to see me he was a 290-pound man in his fifties. I lectured him earnestly on the importance of making time for exercise, but this didn't persuade him to join a gym. His chief complaints were high cholesterol, high blood pressure, imbalanced blood-sugar levels, and frequent headaches. His family history was laden with heart complications and diabetes, so this was exactly where he was headed if it wasn't already too late. I almost told him that I wouldn't take his case because I felt that there would be no compliance on his end. He promised that he would take anything I recommended or eat any way I suggested, but he wouldn't have time to exercise.

I took his blood pressure that day and found it to be a dangerous 192/94; he was already taking three medications. I explained that his high blood pressure was causing his headaches and that he needed to get re-evaluated by his doctor. His body impedance analysis revealed a body mass index of 41, a total body fat percentage of 46, a metabolic rate of 2,300 calories and a significant retention of water. I screened him for free radical levels, and he was 4 of 5 on the colorimetric urine MDA analysis. I started him on magnesium, alpha-lipoic acid, CoQ_{10}, vitamins A, E and D and a high dose B-complex. I outlined a diet for him amounting to 2,000 calories per day worth of ORAC-only foods for the highest concentration of antioxidant power. I saw him again in four months (he was too busy to make three interim appointments), and to my delight he had lost fifty pounds. His body impedance analysis revealed that forty-three of those lost pounds were specifically fat tissue.

When I congratulated him, I suggested that if he kept the weight off he could probably add three years onto his life expectancy. When I asked if he had complied with all that I had asked him to do, he reported that he had taken the antioxidants for the first month but hadn't realized he was supposed to do so on an ongoing basis. On re-evaluation, his urine MDA levels were down to 2 out of 5. While he was not out of the woods yet, and needed to be on a therapeutic antioxidant routine for some time to come, he had essentially lost fifty pounds in four months and reduced a huge free radical load by simply eating a diet of high ORAC-value foods. He was most happy that he didn't have to give up his one morning coffee, a small piece of dark chocolate and the one glass of red wine a day the diet allowed.

FURTHER RESEARCH RESOURCES AND HOME TESTING KITS

For a complete listing of the books, articles and research studies I relied on for *The Antioxidant Prescription*, please visit my website at www.drwylde.com. In case you wish to do further research online, the following are researchers, companies or organizations that I have found to be both groundbreaking and scientifically reliable.

RESEARCHERS

Dr. Bruce Ames
www.bruceames.org

Dr. Denham Harman
www.nebraska.edu/about/pioneers.asp?p=27

Dr. Lester Packer www.pharmanex.com/corp/pharmanews/sab/lester_packer
.shtml

Dr. Joe McCord www.protandim.com/Default.aspx?Page=
LifeVantageCorporation

Dr. Leonard Hayflick
www.mpib-berlin.mpg.de/en/aktuelles/hayflick.htm

Dr. Kenneth Cooper
www.cooperaerobics.com

Dr. Andrew Weil
www.drweil.com

Dr. Michael Colgan
www.colganinstitute.com

SUPPLEMENT COMPANIES

Metagenics
(Leaders in medical food and vitamin/mineral formulas)
www.metagenics.com

Ascenta
(Leaders in fish oil)
www.ascentahealth.com

Advanced Orthomolecular Research (AOR)
(Leaders in antioxidants)
www.aor.ca

Boiron
(Leaders in homeopathic dilutions)
www.boiron.com

Heel Canada
(Leaders in homotoxicology)
www.heel.ca

Cold-fX
(Leaders in cold and flu solutions)
www.coldfx.com

FOOD

Nimbus Water Systems
(Water services, specializing in reverse osmosis water)
www.nimbuswater.com

NutritionData
(Everything from calories to quality)
www.nutritiondata.com

FitDay
(Free nutrition analysis and journal)
www.fitday.com

Fruits & Veggies More Matters
(How many per day?)
www.fruitsandveggiesmorematters.org

Seafood Selector
(Toxicities in seafood)
www.oceansalive.org/eat.cfm?subnav=healthalerts

Center for Science in the Public Interest
(From eating green to food safety issues)
www.cspinet.org

Food Safety
(U.S. government food safety information)
www.foodsafety.gov
(Canadian government food safety information)
www.hc-sc.gc.ca/fn-an/securit/index.html

LifeWare
(Healthy cookware)
www.lifeware.us

World Health Organization on Nutrition
http://www.who.int/nutrition/en/

USDA Center for Nutrition Policy and Promotion
www.usda.gov/cnpp/

Environmental Defence
www.environmentaldefence.ca

PRODUCTS AND SERVICES

Hyperhealth
(Nutrition and natural health database)
www.hyperhealth.com

Healthnotes
www.healthnotes.com

Healthfinder
(Health information from U.S. Department of Health and Human Services)
www.healthfinder.gov

Life Extension Foundation
www.lef.org

Skin Deep
(Cosmetic safety database by Environmental Working Group)
www.cosmeticsdatabase.com

Guide to Less Toxic Products
www.lesstoxicguide.ca

Pollution Information
(U.S. information)
www.scorecard.org/env-releases/land

Household Toxin Reduction
(How to create a healthy home)
www.lowtox.com

Ecological and Non-Toxic Paint
www.ecopaints.co.uk *and* www.eartheasy.com/live_nontoxic_paints.htm

SAD Lights
(Light therapy)
www.litebook.com

Nozone
(UV protective clothing)
http://www.nozone.ca/

ConsumerLab
(Keeping manufacturers of natural medicines accountable)
www.consumerlab.com

ClinicalTrials
(Recent trials on antioxidants)
www.clinicaltrials.gov (key "antioxidants" in search command)

Cantox
(Regulatory consulting firm specializing in food and nutrition)
www.cantox.com

Radon House Gas Services
Canada: http://gsc.nrcan.gc.ca/gamma/radon_e.php
USA: www.epa.gov/ebtpages/pollradiatradon.html

GOVERNMENT, UNIVERSITY AND OTHER AGENCIES

Environment Canada
http://www.on.ec.gc.ca/or-home.html

U.S. Environmental Protection Agency
www.epa.gov

Environmental Defence Canada
www.environmentaldefence.ca

Environmental Science and Technology
http://pubs.acs.org/journals/esthag/index.html

Agency for Toxic Substances and Disease Registry
(U.S. Department of Health and Human Services)
www.atsdr.cdc.gov

Safe Wireless Initiative
www.safewireless.org

How Mercury Causes Brain Neuron Degeneration (video)
http://commons.ucalgary.ca/mercury/

Centers for Disease Control and Prevention: Skin Cancer
www.cdc.gov/cancer/skin

Integrated Risk Information System: Bisphenol A
http://www.epa.gov/iris/subst/0356.htm

Life Without Plastic
(Glass and stainless steel bottles and other non-plastic items)
www.lifewithoutplastic.com

ORAC Watch
http://www.oracwatch.org/

Free Radical Biology & Medicine
(Journal of the Society for Free Radical Biology and Medicine)
www.elsevier.com/locate/freeradbiomed

Pacific Northwest National Laboratory
(Free radical science and research lab)
www.sysbio.org/sysbio/stress/

Oxis International Inc.
(Develops technologies and products to research, diagnose, treat and prevent diseases of oxidative stress)
www.oxis.com

Society for Free Radical Biology and Medicine
sfrbm.org/index.cfm

Sunrise Free Radical Biology and Medicine School
www.healthcare.uiowa.edu/research/sfrbm/

Society for Free Radical Research—Europe
www.sfrr-europe.org

U.S. National Cancer Institute
Antioxidants and Cancer Prevention: Fact Sheet
http://www.cancer.gov/cancertopics/factsheet/antioxidantsprevention

The Institute for Functional Medicine
www.functionalmedicine.org

LABORATORIES

Neurosciences Lab., Inc.
www.neurorelicf.com

Genox Corporation
www.genox.com

Genova Diagnostics
www.gdx.net/home

Brunswick Laboratories
www.brunswicklabs.com

Gemoscan International, Inc.
www.gemoscan.com

Cayman Chemical
www.caymanchem.com

OXIS International, Inc.
www.oxis.com/biocheck.html

HOME TESTING

Bryce Wylde's Antioxidant Test Kit was discussed at some length in Chapter Five. It is a simple series of three non-invasive urine tests that will assist you in determining the free radical levels in your body, and help determine the effectiveness of your diet, and perhaps more importantly the effectiveness of any vitamins or supplements that you may be taking—so as to empower you as a consumer to "debunk the junk"

I am extending an invitation here to those who have purchased my book to purchase my free radical test kit at a reduced rate. The offer can be found along with an order form on the last page of this book. Simply fill out the form and mail it to the address indicated, or order online at **www.drwylde.com**, using the promotional discount code printed on the order form.

I maintain a private e-health newsletter for my patients that aims to assist them in keeping up to the moment with the evolving scientific literature on antioxidants and free radicals. I invite readers of *The Antioxidant Prescription* to enroll in this email newsletter membership for free on my website by checking the appropriate box on the test kit order form.

ACKNOWLEDGEMENTS

To this point, few people other than scientists have been able to interpret the impact of free radicals in human disease. I am honoured to be one of the few authors to bring this information to you in an understandable and applicable form so that you may use it to thwart disease, to live longer and healthier lives. However, I could never have done this myself. I give credit and sincere thanks to my substantive editor, Robert Buckland, for his ingenious ability to turn my scientific language into readable yet accurate prose. He is truly gifted.

This work has many other incredible people behind it. I would like to express my gratitude to Anne Collins, the publisher of Random House Canada, for her commitment to this project and her belief in me right from the beginning. If it weren't for you, all of this would have remained a dream. Heartfelt appreciation also must go to my literary agent, John Pearce, for his diligence in seeing the possibilities and properly managing my expectations! Thank you to Cory Pala, for being a true friend, exceptional sounding board and formidable business partner. A shout-out to Mike Day of "The Art of Weddings" who took my cover shot (since we *loved* our wedding photos, I figured Mike could do as good a job on a cover photo). Lastly, my true thanks to Scott Richardson, the creative director of Random House Canada, for getting the look of this book just right.

Special thanks to my good friends and colleagues, Bruce Krahn and Teresa Tapp. Your contributions make the exercise chapter of this book an excellent one. My muscles and my waistline already thank you, and I'm sure my readers' will too.

It took years to research this book, not only in the scientific literature but in the hectic to-and-fro of a practice where I've treated thousands of patients according to the ideas in this book. But I believe that my efforts here pale in comparison to the dedication and effort my mother, Primrose Anne, devoted to single-handedly raising me and my two sisters as healthy, happy and grounded people. She has always been ahead of her time, and her example is my guiding light in spreading the message of wellness. To my father, Darryl, thanks for the genetics required to spend countless nights up until 3 a.m. in the grip of an obsession and for your support in getting me through school.

To Tanya, my little sister, who is a naturopathic doctor and my clinic associate: I plan to work side by side with you forever— or at least until we've convinced the world that these principles of healing and health are correct. My older sister Julie is a teacher extraordinaire, with enough life experience to give anyone the lessons of a lifetime. To Eve, for your constant support and equally constant kvetching; to Abe for your unconditional love and remaining oblivious to the fact that I'd written a book until you read these words! To Peter Weleff and family: thank you for being there for me through my childhood years and helping me to realize how invaluable it would be to become a professional. Rhonda, Sandra, Mike, Carly, Alison, Eden, Jayden, Skylar and Cameron—your names are here because of how much I love you all.

To my Aunt June, a warm and gentle soul, who passed away while I was writing this book: we all love you and miss you. My aunt's devotion to taking her antioxidants during her battle against breast cancer helped her to live long past her prognosis.

To Devin and Zaya, my children and my reasons for being. I know you don't like Daddy so much when he "taints" your water and juice with all those antioxidants, vitamins and essential oils, and tricks you with organic carob instead of chocolate, but I hope you'll thank me for it later. I'm following in my mother's footsteps!

Last, but never least, my deepest gratitude is to my beautiful wife, Kelly. Without your support, your love for natural medicine and nutrition, and your wonderful self, I couldn't have conceived of doing this project. If it weren't for you, our family would often fail to eat as healthily! Sometimes I can express all that you mean to me in words, but other times even the dictionary falls short. You were created in part to stump the dictionary.

Love, peace and especially good health to you all!

INDEX

Page numbers in **boldface** refer to material discussed in charts and tables.

BRYCE WYLDE'S ANTIOXIDANT TEST KIT—ORDER FORM

Save 20% on introductory test kit—Includes FREE 2nd test set to monitor progress

Order online at www.drwylde.com (enter promotional code: AP1408). Or mail or fax completed form to:

Bryce Wylde Testing
P.O. Box 66, Station A
Toronto, Ontario M5W 1A2
Toll Free: 1–800–960–6046
FAX: (416) 981–7477

Visa, Mastercard, cheque or money order only
Make cheques payable to:
Wylde Pala Enterprises Inc.

DESCRIPTION

Bryce Wylde Free Radical Test Kit $99.99 (less 20% promotion) $79.99

Includes: *One Free Radical Test*
               One Stress (Adrenal) Test
               One Vitamin C Test

Bonus included is a 2nd Test Set for Follow-up Treatment Monitoring ***FREE!***

Unit Quantity _____ X $79.99 = $ _____

GST (5%) Canadians Only ($4.00 per kit) $ _____

Shipping and Handling
($8.00 Canada; $14.00 Outside Canada) $ _____

Total Payable $ _____   ***International orders contact***
(Outside Canada all prices in U.S. dollars)   ***distribution@drwylde.com***

PLEASE PRINT CLEARLY   ***Outside Canada all prices in U.S. dollars***

NAME: _____

ADDRESS: _____

CITY & PROVINCE/STATE: _____ POSTAL/ZIP CODE:_____

HOME PHONE: (_____) ___ _____
WORK PHONE: (_____) _____

VISA/MASTERCARD #: _____ EXPIRY DATE: (MM/YY): _____
CVN #___ *
*CVN is a 3-digit code located on the back of your credit card, on the signature strip just to the right of the card number.

SIGNATURE: _____
DATE: _____

EMAIL: _____ (Include for shipping confirmation/tracking)

Please allow 2 to 4 weeks for order processing and delivery
☐ "Yes! I wish to receive Dr. Bryce Wylde's free e-health email reports!"